Praise for *Healing Adaptogens*

"For decades I've been a fan of functional mushrooms and modulating herbs, also known as Adaptogens. They are some of the most underrated, yet powerful, tools for metabolic health, performance, and longevity.Tero, and this book, are an excellent entryway to learn how you can leverage them in your daily life."

— Mark Hyman, M.D., 14x *New York Times* best-selling author

"As a functional medicine expert, I have been a longtime fan of Adaptogens, but most of the information out there is confusing and difficult to wade through. Never before has there been such a comprehensive and easy to understand resource for those looking to take advantage of the healing power of Adaptogens. From the most popular Adaptogens, their numerous health benefits, where to buy them, and exactly how to use them, Tero makes it easier than ever to harness these often overlooked and misunderstood plant and herbal medicines for your health."

— Dr. Will Cole, leading functional medicine expert, IFMCP, DNM, DC, host of *The Art Of Being Well*, and author of *Ketotarian, The Inflammation Spectrum*, and *New York Times* bestseller, *Intuitive Fasting*

"Finally, a comprehensive and accessible go-to guide on Adaptogens! For anyone who's heard the word but still doesn't truly understand how they work, this book is for you. Tero and Danielle offer a fun and easy-to-follow guide on these powerful super herbs and functional mushrooms. This is the book to help guide you toward a life of less stress, stronger immunity, sharper mental and physical performance, and an overall upgrade in your day-to-day wellbeing. Absolutely a must-read!"

— Kelly LeVeque, celebrity nutritionist and best-selling author

"This book takes head-on the important but complex concept of adaptogens. It does a masterful job in introducing why this family of plant nutrients are so important in establishing health through promoting balance in how our bodies work. This book provides a guide for those who want to incorporate the power of plant adaptogens as a tool in achieving optimal health."

— Jeffrey Bland, Ph.D., president of Personalized Lifestyle Medicine Institute

"Danielle is one of my go-to leaders in Adaptogens, herbs, and mushrooms. In this book, she has taken all her knowledge and condensed it in order to help us, the readers, understand the scientific benefit behind many of these popular health ingredients. No marketing jargon, just the facts about some of the most powerful herbs and agents out there. So happy that Danielle has provided this guide for everyone from a health & wellness advocate to a seasoned practitioner. Thanks, Danielle!"

— Christian Gonzalez, N.D., Integrative Oncology, Chronic Disease & General Medicine

"Healing Adaptogens is a fantastic book on the benefits of these powerful super herbs and functional mushrooms. We finally have a definite guide in the functional benefits of Adaptogens. Tero makes learning about them easy and fun. If you're interested in being the best and healthiest version of yourself, this is a must-read!"

— Dhru Purohit, entrepreneur, investor, and podcast host

"From the Chaga filled forests of Finland to the shores of North America, Tero shines a light on the complex and fascinating world of Adaptogens and the beneficial role that functional mushrooms play. He and Danielle also demystify the extraction methods and quality issues that are essential to choosing top quality supplements. Highly recommended."

— Jeff Chilton, mushroom expert and founder of Nammex

"Healing Adaptogens is a practical guide to helping anyone feel and perform better, both mentally and physically. Easy to understand and implement, I recommend this book to everyone I know who feels the strain of modern life, which is everyone I know. The advice works and is a long-term solution to burnout. It's an investment in your future."

— Brendan Brazier, best-selling author and co-founder of Vega and Pulp Culture

"Adaptogens are a truly remarkable category within human nutrition. Today, when stress-related illnesses are at an all-time high, the education and utilization of adaptogens is more important than ever. Thankfully, we have a valuable guide available to us all in Healing Adaptogens."

— Shawn Stevenson, author of *USA Today* best-selling book *Eat Smarter* and international best-selling book *Sleep Smarter*

HEALING
ADAPTOGENS

HEALING
ADAPTOGENS

The Definitive Guide to Using Super
Herbs and Mushrooms for Your
Body's Restoration, Defence
and Performance

Tero Isokauppila
Founder of Four Sigmatic®

Danielle Ryan Broida
RH (AHG)

HAY HOUSE

Carlsbad, California • New York City
London • Sydney • New Delhi

Published in the United Kingdom by:
Hay House UK Ltd, The Sixth Floor, Watson House,
54 Baker Street, London W1U 7BU
Tel: +44 (0)20 3927 7290; Fax: +44 (0)20 3927 7291; www.hayhouse.co.uk

Published in the United States of America by:
Hay House Inc., PO Box 5100, Carlsbad, CA 92018-5100
Tel: (1) 760 431 7695 or (800) 654 5126
Fax: (1) 760 431 6948 or (800) 650 5115; www.hayhouse.com

Published in Australia by:
Hay House Australia Ltd, 18/36 Ralph St, Alexandria NSW 2015
Tel: (61) 2 9669 4299; Fax: (61) 2 9669 4144; www.hayhouse.com.au

Published in India by:
Hay House Publishers India, Muskaan Complex, Plot No.3, B-2,
Vasant Kunj, New Delhi 110 070
Tel: (91) 11 4176 1620; Fax: (91) 11 4176 1630; www.hayhouse.co.in

Indexer: J S Editorial, LLC
Cover design: The Book Designers
Interior design: Bryn Starr Best
Interior illustrations: Juho Heinola

A catalogue record for this book is available from the British Library.

Tradepaper ISBN: 978-1-78817-729-0
Printed Paper Cased ISBN: 978-1-4019-6674-4
E-book ISBN: 978-1-4019-6675-1
Audiobook ISBN: 978-1-4019-6676-8

This product uses papers sourced from responsibly managed forests. For more information, see www.hayhouse.co.uk.

Printed and bound by CPI Group (UK) Ltd, Croydon, CR0 4YY

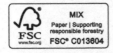

We dedicate this book
to Pachamama,
intergalactic spores,
and Dr. Nikolai Lazarev.

CONTENTS

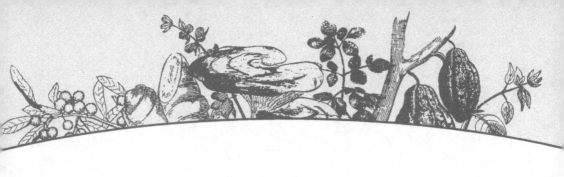

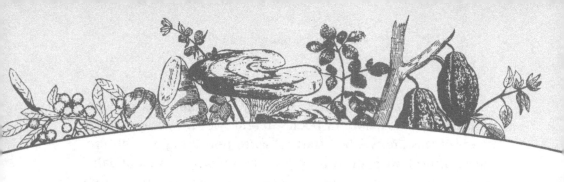

INTRODUCTION

Your alarm sounds. Exhausted, you hit snooze—twice. By the time you get out of bed, you're already behind. You make a big cup of coffee to combat the brain fog, likely from the wine last night. You get a bit jittery from it, but it's better than feeling foggy. You wash down a bowl of sugary cereal with another cup of coffee. By midday, you start to crash. Time for the third cup of caffeine, maybe in the form of an energy drink, and a granola bar. By the end of the day, you're exhausted, but the caffeine and sugar are keeping you wired.

Unfortunately, there's still more to do: dinner, house chores, and personal care. By the time you finish, it feels like you've completed a marathon. You deserve a reward. You're also on a second or third wind, so you need something to cool off and tell your nervous system that you're finally done for the day. A glass of wine fits the bill. Eventually, a little tipsy, you head to bed. You're tired but wired; half asleep, half awake. The night goes by without the depth of sleep your body needs. You wake up groggy. Wash, rinse, repeat.

The most common unifying experience in modern life is stress, and it's taking a serious toll on our health.[1] To cope, it's easy to rely on hyperpalatable food, alcohol, and pharmaceuticals. Yet we are not getting better. The tools we are using to cope are keeping our mental and physical energy low, prohibiting us from sleeping well, and causing us to perform at only the level of merely scraping by.

With this unhealthy cycle so many of us are stuck in, we're not making it easy for our bodies to *deal* with the compounding stress of this lifestyle. For starters, we're not eating enough produce. Instead, we're overeating processed foods, meat, and dairy. Plus, we're consuming more calories than ever before. A 2021 peer-reviewed study concluded that 67 percent of calories young people consume come from ultra-processed foods such as chips, cookies, frozen pizza, and burgers.[2]

Of the few healthy foods we do eat, a lot of them are grown in soil that isn't as nutrient-rich as it was 100 years ago. In fact, the nutrient density of the 43 most common fruits and vegetables has declined.[3] So even when we are eating clean, our bodies have fewer tools to bring us back to a state of balance.

If you are anything like most Americans, there are also several pharmaceuticals thrown into the mix. If one of the causes of stress is an unhealthy diet or nutrient-deficient food, popping a pill may seem like a simple and efficient way to deal with it. Yet despite increased investment in the healthcare industry,[4] we remain sick and stressed.

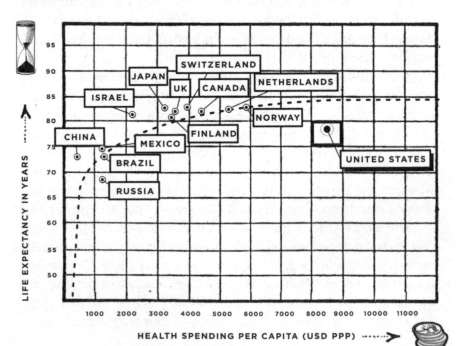

But what if there were another way? A way that shifts your destructive cycle of stress to one of optimized energy, productivity, and balance. A state where *you feel healthy, active, vibrant, and full of life*. One that not only has hundreds of years of traditional wisdom behind it but is also backed by modern science.

Now imagine waking up from a deep night of restful sleep. Your eyes open before the alarm sounds. You have energy, your mind feels clear, and your day is unwritten but full of purpose. You walk into the kitchen and pour yourself a cup of functional coffee. A brew that delivers the full, bold coffee flavor you've known and loved for decades, but this time without the crash, jitters, or upset stomach.

This cup is filled with ancient herbs and mushrooms, ingredients you now leverage to show up as your best self despite the stress of modern-day life. To-dos seamlessly fall off your list as you find time to move your body, engage in activities that bring you pleasure, and spend quality time with your loved ones.

With your newfound state of being, anything off-kilter is painfully noticeable. When an alert triggers stress, you notice your heart pound, palms dampen, and mind race—responses that used to be so familiar. But now, you take a few deep breaths, and just as quickly as that sneaky stressor came, it's gone. You mix another soothing beverage, this time made from Turmeric and other ancient herbs.

As the day rolls on, you move through life like a wave, keenly aware of the chaos around you, yet strong, graceful, and moving with clarity and purpose. You're balanced in a way you once didn't know you were capable of. When the sun sets and dinner is cleaned up, you start the unwinding routine. Just as habitual as your functional coffee is your evening pot of warm Cacao. Your kids still call it hot chocolate, but you know how different it is from the old stuff. This, like your morning brew, is teeming with rich nutrition, delivering the nutrients your whole family needs to start relaxing and preparing for the night's reset.

You pour everyone a mug of this decadent chocolaty treat and sit back smiling, watching as everyone shares stories from their day. When the mugs are dry, your body tells you it's time for rest. Your body effortlessly recedes into sleep, refueling every cell in your body for the day to come.

Welcome to life with Adaptogens. *Adapt-o-what?* In short, the most nutrient-dense, time-tested, ancient natural medicines from around the world. They just happen to be incredibly safe, non-toxic, and for the first time in thousands of years, available and accessible almost anywhere you shop.

ADAPTOGENS IN A NUTSHELL (FOR NOW)

While you may not be familiar with the term "Adaptogens," they have likely been a regular part of your life in some way, shape, or form.

Four Sigmatic has become known for creating the original mushroom coffee, but there's far more to Adaptogens than that! In Chapter 1, we'll fully explore the science of Adaptogens. But for now, you just need to know that they are a group of super plants and functional mushrooms with health benefits, namely helping you *adapt* to all kinds of stressors and situations.

Super plants are medicinal plants that have been used for centuries for their range of benefits to human health. They include some familiar species such as Turmeric and Cacao and more niche ingredients (to Westerners) like Astragalus and Gynostemma. In every culture across the globe, humans have relied on plant medicines to maintain health and ward off sickness. Super plants have a wide range of uses, phytochemicals, and benefits. They help us with energy, stress, mental function, immunity, and more.

Functional mushrooms are a subset of mushrooms in the fungi kingdom that have beneficial effects on human health. If you hear "mushrooms" and think of portobellos on a pizza, we have news for you! Fungi are actually their own biological kingdom, like the plant and animal kingdoms. Out of the millions of species in the fungi kingdom, there are around 700 species that have been used across the world for their medicinal benefits. They are among the most complex, medicinally potent, and yet safest natural medicines on the planet. Many have been used for thousands of years in traditional systems of medicine.

THE BREAKDOWN

Together, we, Danielle and Tero, have helped bring our deep passion and expertise in all things Adaptogens to millions of people seeking health benefits around the world. While doing that, we have had the unique privilege to learn deeply about the sourcing and preparation of these powerful functional foods.

We believe it is important to source ingredients from their native lands whenever possible. We also feel it's critically important to source ingredients in their most authentic form—the way they are found in nature and the way our ancestors have been using them for millennia.

While we don't take ourselves too seriously, our dedication to finding the highest quality ingredients possible is no joke. We taste, test, and experiment with every single ingredient to find the highest quality and most authentic options out there. We feel humbled to be a small part of reviving these Adaptogens, bringing them to the Western palate, where people truly need the benefits they offer. We acknowledge that we are standing on the shoulders of giants with many ancient cultures, scientists, and amazing herbal educators to thank. We honor that these plants and mushrooms have been part of the fabric of health in societies across the world and hope to keep their magic alive by offering them in a practical way to the West.

While ancient intent is a powerful basis to work from, the current world and our stress levels require a comprehensive approach that integrates traditional knowledge with modern research.

Our philosophy about optimal, sustained health is rooted in long-term solutions rather than bandages. We believe our bodies are wise and desire to not just survive but to *thrive*.

Think of your health as a flowing river. There are often obstacles—dams or boulders—preventing the river from flowing smoothly. In our bodies, these obstructions are stress, nutrient deficiencies, and a reliance on unhealthy coping mechanisms. When we remove the obstacles, the river can flow freely again.

Adaptogens are our river keepers, helping to remove obstacles so our health is no longer obstructed from showing up in full vitality. They help get our bodies back into a state of balance and health. They safely support our body's energy to move like a free-flowing river—not just today or tomorrow, but when we're 90 and beyond. After all, the stressors of modern-day are likely not going away anytime soon. Knowing this, we need to become more adaptable and more "anti-fragile"!

OUR ADAPTOGEN ORIGIN STORIES

Tero Isokauppila

Tero's path to learning and sharing the power of natural healing started at his family farm in Finland. In Finland, saunas outnumber cars, and people love coffee as much as they love nature. The Isokauppilas have been taking care of their land in southern Finland near the town of Nokia (yep, famous for the mobile phones) since around 1619. Tero and his brother, Vesa, make up the thirteenth generation in the family to care for this land, and their young sons, Banyan and Antti, will be the fourteenth.

Tero's father is an agronomist, and his mother taught physiology and anatomy to nurses. Growing up in Finland, Tero learned to appreciate the best off-the-beaten-track ingredients and the absolute worst puns. He also developed an appreciation for both the power of earth and science, scientist and farmer, slow and fast, and ancient and modern. Following this bridged path, Tero went on to study chemistry, nutrition, and business in the USA, Canada, the UK, France, and Finland. But when he left the farm, he realized that not everyone's grandparents brewed a coffee replacement made from Chaga during WWII.

In 2012, Tero started Four Sigmatic to share these powerful Finnish traditions with the world. With friends and colleagues, Tero searched around the world for exhaustively studied, practically magical Adaptogens that could be added to people's daily staples. He wanted to help people create better *daily routines* that incorporate ancient wild foods, including mushrooms and other plant Adaptogens. Tero has spent the last 15 years living in 10 countries, pioneering the functional mushroom and Adaptogen space.

Danielle Ryan Broida

Danielle's story began on the other side of the world in Southern California, which is quite the opposite of freezing Finland. California life looked dreamy from the outside, but within her hometown of Montecito, she could see that incredible wealth, fame, and access weren't enough to shield people from ill health, stress, and depression. This led her to seek a deeper understanding of sustainable happiness and health from a very early age.

After receiving her B.A. in environmental studies and philosophy from Whitman College, Danielle moved to Southeast Asia to learn about the environment, traditional medicine, and alternative healing from the source. She ended up studying Ayurvedic medicine in India, becoming a certified Ashtanga and Hatha yoga instructor on the banks of the Ganges River, and studying under a naturopathic doctor in Indonesia, where she became a certified raw chef and detox coach. But it was leading trekking adventures into the backcountry of Thailand where she became particularly fascinated by herbal medicine while also becoming fluent in Thai. She then began to follow traditional ways of living, focusing primarily on wild and natural foods and medicines.

Danielle returned to the United States to formalize her graduate education in holistic medicine at the Colorado School of Clinical Herbalism. She went on to open a private clinical practice, where she focused on functional mushroom-based treatment for autoimmune conditions and chronic illnesses. She has worked with hundreds of clients, supporting their journeys to health and vitality with the help of herbal and fungal medicine. After several years in clinical practice, she became a Registered Herbalist of the American Herbalists Guild. She now teaches at CSCH as their instructor of mycology while being Tero's partner in education at Four Sigmatic.

WHY *HEALING ADAPTOGENS* WAS WRITTEN

We designed this book to help you easily navigate when, how, and why to use Adaptogens. We've combined traditional wisdom with the most up-to-date research on these magical herbs and fungi to create a practical and comprehensive guide. We wrote this book because it didn't exist. The Internet is full of blogs with bullet points on various Adaptogens, and while some have valid facts, most are just marketing. There are a handful of great clinical books and resources about the science behind Adaptogens that are full of quality information, but these clinical texts can be hard to read and tend to focus on one or a limited number of Adaptogens, lack a description of how to use and buy Adaptogens, or are outdated.

We've both been studying Adaptogens for over a decade. This book is the definitive yet playful guidebook we wish had existed when we started on this path.

HOW TO READ AND USE THIS BOOK

This book is focused on the top 21 Adaptogens, dividing them into three main categories: **Defend, Perform**, and **Restore**.

Since by definition, Adaptogens cannot be boxed into a specific singular benefit, it can become confusing how and why to start using them. We created this categorization to give you a starting place for when and why to use each one. Adaptogens to Defend are those best for immune support and beauty, Adaptogens to Perform are for energy and focus, and Adaptogens to Restore are for stress and longevity.

But before we get too deep into the benefits, stories, and use cases of the Adaptogens themselves, we need to lay the foundation for your journey.

PART I will guide you through the discovery of Adaptogens, what they are, the science behind how they work, how they interact with key systems of your body, and how to choose the right Adaptogen for your unique body and needs.

PART II dives into the ingredients, the Adaptogens themselves. Each of the 21 profiles focuses on an individual Adaptogen to give you the confidence to know when and why to bring that Adaptogen into your routine, its key benefits, and even how to vet the highest quality products to receive the best results.

PART III starts with a shopping guide, because this book would not be the practical guide we set out to create without tips and tricks on how to start using (which first entails purchasing) these healing Adaptogens for whole-body health. We give you information on what to look for when buying Adaptogens (warning: there's unfortunately a ton of shady marketing around Adaptogens) and share multiple commonly available and small business options on where to buy them.

Then we provide you with our 10 Commandments of Adaptogens to provide an easy, go-to reference for their daily usage, which we follow with tips for realistically and sustainably integrating Adaptogens into your everyday routine.

The end of the book includes our endnotes and an index. While these don't seem like the sexiest parts of the book, we encourage you to use them to help you navigate the text and use as a source to refer to for years to come. Just like the fact boxes at the start of each Adaptogen profile, the index helps you save time. Head straight there if you're looking for a specific term or need, or skim through it to find interesting parts about the book for your limited reading time.

Once you've read the book once or twice, you'll find the scientific references are an excellent place to dive even deeper and continue your learning journey. We have carefully read through over one thousand studies, and these select references can save you time when looking for valuable insights. We have ignored many weaker sources and focused on the better-designed (double-blind, placebo-controlled, and peer-reviewed) references, when possible.

We truly hope this book is just the beginning of your journey with Adaptogens. The real fun starts when you close the book and experience these powerful plants and mushrooms in your own life. Danielle often tells her clients, "Don't just trust me . . . experience the Adaptogens for yourself because the relationship with each plant or mushroom begins with you."

This can be thought of like matchmaking. You are pairing yourself, a unique being (one that is also constantly changing!) with another whole being (in the form of a super plant or functional mushroom). The relationship you forge with that species will be yours and yours alone. So get on with it—go do some dating with Adaptogens!

As you play and experiment with these ingredients that for thousands of years were only for the elite, wildly expensive, or prayed over as sacred, please remember to take care of yourself. To be safe with experimentation, especially if you have a health condition or are taking medications, always check in with your healthcare practitioner before taking any new supplements, including Adaptogens.

We feel humbled and fortunate to have these ingredients at our fingertips today, arguably the time when we need these allies the most. Let this book be the bridge between where you are now and the life of waking up each day as the best, most vital version of yourself. May this be your reference guide and a place you come back to time and again as you move through your Adaptogenic journey. Onward!

PART I

THE
SCIENCE
OF
ADAPTOGENS

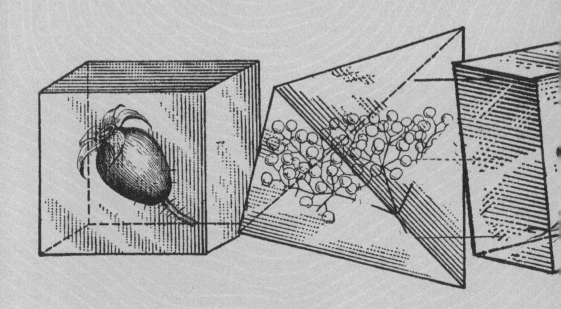

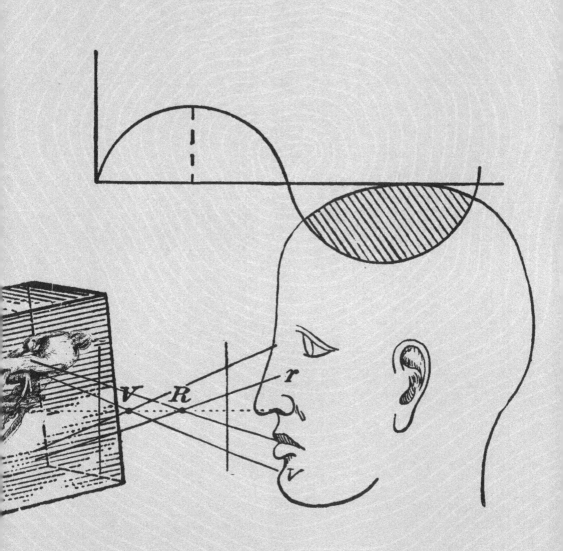

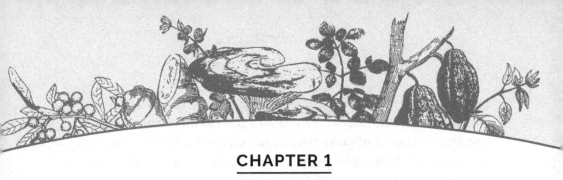

CHAPTER 1

DEFINING ADAPTOGENS

Take a moment to think of your body as a city. Cities have reservoirs to pull water from in times of need. Similarly, think of your body having its own reservoir, a "vital reserve." If you encounter drought, a stressor, you can pull from the reservoir to keep the taps flowing and the people of your city, or cells, replenished.

Adaptogens help replenish your vital reserve so that when stressors arise (which is inevitable), there is a pool of resources to draw from. This enables your body to respond to the stressor efficiently and return to a state of balance efficiently.

WHAT MAKES AN ADAPTOGEN

All Adaptogens must meet three criteria to qualify as a true Adaptogen.

First, they must be **nontoxic**. This means they have minimal side effects. There is no "toxic load" where taking too much will push you over the edge and lead to negative consequences. Instead, there is merely a "ceiling dose." This means that once you take up to a certain amount, the benefits will plateau, as your body cannot utilize more than a given amount. There are many plants that have wonderful health applications (like *Bryonia alba*, or wild hops, for example), so they might be considered a superfood, but their toxic load excludes them from the Adaptogenic category.

Second, they must be **nonspecific**. This is where much of the confusion with Adaptogens arises. Unlike most other medicines, they do not push your body in one direction or another. Instead, they build adaptive energy in your body, rather than exert a specific effect like stimulation or relaxation. This mechanism occurs through a range of phytonutrients that effects multiple systems in the body to encourage balance. Most natural and pharmaceutical medicines have a specific action. Examples in plants include *Passiflora incarnata* (passionflower), which directly sedates your body, or *Camellia sinensis* (green or black tea), which stimulates it.

Lastly, to qualify as an Adaptogen, the species must have a **normalizing** effect. This is seen through normalizing systems including the immune, endocrine, nervous, cardiovascular, and digestive systems. Normalizing means there is a bidirectional effect on physiological function. Adaptogens often contain compounds with opposing effects. These are compounds that work synergistically in Adaptogens that, if isolated, act quite differently. The same ingredient can be energizing or relaxing, and the compound needed to bring your body into a state of balance will have a "louder" effect than others. Think of them as calibrators, adapting to each body's unique needs. We like to think of this as a gas-brake effect.

An example of the gas-brake effect can be seen in Cacao. This incredible bean has many compounds, two of which are relevant to call out here: theobromine, which has a gas effect, and magnesium, which has a braking effect. Depending on the person who consumes Cacao, it may either elevate their energy or allow them to rest deeper. Cacao adapts its action to bring your body into a *normalized* or balanced state.

Let's look at a visual representation of how Adaptogens normalize your body in response to stressors.

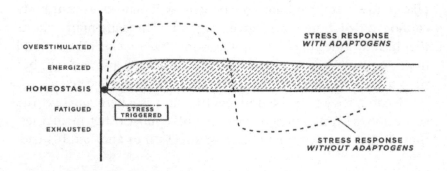

In the graph, you can visually see Adaptogens' stress-protective effect. The dotted line is your body's typical response to a stressor. The solid line is your body's response to that same stressful event with the support of Adaptogens. The solid line never drops below the line of *homeostasis*. Homeostasis is the body's rhythmic calibrator that continuously interacts and adjusts with changes within or outside the body. It allows us to function in a stable manner, keeping the body within a set range of normal parameters, including blood pressure, heart rate, temperature, and more. Instead of significantly rocking the body out of this set parameter of homeostasis, with Adaptogens on board, the body slowly is relieved of the initial stressor and returns to a state of homeostasis without ever being depleted to the point of fatigue and exhaustion.

Without Adaptogens, your body is on a roller coaster. It's quickly stimulated, spiking in its hormonal and endocrinal response to a state of high alert, followed by an energy crash, and eventually exhaustion. With Adaptogens, the body uses less energy to respond to the perceived stressor. It does not immediately go into a phase of high alert but rather is slightly elevated in acuity. The gentle stimulating effect also lasts longer. The key here is that with Adaptogens on board, the body does not crash and require a phase of exhaustion before bouncing back to homeostasis.

THROUGH THE LENS OF TRADITIONAL MEDICINE

As humans, we have relied on plants as medicine for thousands of years. Long before they were "discovered" and categorized as Adaptogens, these same species were used in cultures across the world. This particular group of plants and mushrooms was especially revered and utilized in traditional systems of medicine, particularly Ayurveda and Traditional Chinese Medicine (TCM). Much of the traditional stories and use cases come from these two systems.

Understanding the philosophy of these systems helps to understand why Adaptogens were revered and used as such prominent species in these cultures. Much of the oldest preserved information and documentation of these species comes from these two lineages. There are many other ancient cultures from Mexico to Scandinavia, the Amazon to Sub-Saharan Africa, who have also used Adaptogens for a long time, but these two happened to document the effects better than other cultures. These systems are comparable to what "Western medicine" is to the United States today.

In these two systems and beyond, these species have been used as currency, food, and medicine. The reemergence of Adaptogens in the West is therefore more of a remembrance. It's a way of looking back at the tools that have helped humans survive through thousands of years of hardship and enabled them to endure long, cold winters (with Rhodiola and Chaga), to keep their immune systems strong (with Eleuthero and Turkey Tail), minds sharp (with Mucuna, Gotu Kola, and Lion's Mane), and bodies in shape (with Cordyceps and Maca).

There are two central differences between Western medicine versus TCM and Ayurveda. First, in the Western system of medicine, the body is viewed as a machine consisting of isolated parts. In TCM and Ayurveda, the body is viewed as an interconnected ecosystem, where one part always affects others. The second difference is the treatment approach. In Western medicine, symptoms are treated. In TCM and Ayurveda, symptoms are merely a temporary expression of an underlying imbalance, and as such, the whole body is treated. TCM and Ayurveda both look at individual body types versus symptoms. In both systems, the body has a unique characteristic (temperament, dosha, or constitution), so the individual, not the ailment, is treated. Western medicine, on the other hand, does not consider individual body types, as that is irrelevant when treating a symptom: a headache is a headache regardless of the body experiencing it. Lastly, in many traditional systems of medicine, doctors get paid if you are healthy, not if you're sick—since that's when they have failed in their job. In Western medicine, the health practitioner gets paid by treating you when you're sick.

This framework sets the stage for how Adaptogens are used in these cultures. They are used to support the whole, individual body rather than a specific condition. A person may be presenting with specific symptoms like restlessness or headaches, but instead of using an Adaptogen to target that symptom, the Adaptogen should be used to replenish and support the foundational systems of the body, so the symptoms can naturally resolve themselves.

While we are forever grateful for the advancements of modern medicine (for example, fixing Tero's ACL after two soccer injuries), Adaptogens are a bit more aligned with the TCM and Ayurvedic philosophies in the way they support your body. Viewing them through a different lens, much like these traditional systems, will help you understand how they work in your body.

TCM

TCM is an acronym for Traditional Chinese Medicine, which is the second-largest system of medicine practiced in the world today. This 3,500-year-old system includes various forms of healing including natural medicine, diet, and several bodywork practices (acupuncture, cupping, massage, gua sha, etc.). TCM focuses on your body's vital energy, called Ch'i or Qi. This vital energy source is believed to circulate throughout your body through channels called meridians. Think of it like blood flow, with more energetic force to it. The meridians have branches that extend to organs, controlling the health of your body's functions. Disease occurs when the Qi is imbalanced or not flowing harmoniously. Thus, treatment of disease in TCM addresses patterns of underlying imbalance.

Ayurveda

In Sanskrit, "Ayur" means "life" or "longevity" and "Veda" means "science" or "sacred knowledge." Ayurveda is the 5,000-year-old holistic healing system of India and the third-largest system of medicine practiced around the world today. In Ayurveda, disease arises from a state of imbalance—mentally, physically, or spiritually. The world's oldest health system, Ayurveda is known as a healing science *and* art, connecting mind and body. It is the foundational science of yoga and focuses on diet, natural medicines, movement, breathwork, and spiritual practices to bring about whole-body health. We can also thank Ayurveda for many of the meditation practices that are popular today.

ENERGETICS: NATURAL MEDICINE MATCHMAKING

You might not have heard of the "energetics" of a plant or mushroom before. In this book, we share the energetics of each species based on its ancient intent. In most traditional systems of medicine, there are categories of body types (known as doshas, temperaments, or constitutions). There was a recognition that not all bodies were the same. Instead, there were groups of body types, often categorized by the elements, temperature, and moisture. The philosophy of a single pill for an ailment is relatively new. Rather than identifying a condition and treating that condition, your body was understood to be a unique ecosystem that required unique care. Since each natural species, plant or fungi, is also a complex and unique being, the process of treating an individual with a natural medicine was a bit like matchmaking.

In Ayurveda, there are three recognized doshas or body types based on the five elements: pitta (fire), vata (air + ether), and kapha (earth + water). Each person contains all three doshic energies within them in varying degrees. The goal is to return to a state where your three doshas are aligned with the ratio they were at when you came into existence (called your 'prakriti dosha'). Herbs and natural medicines were also grouped into categories. There was an understanding that not all medicines were created equal because some are moist (such as aloe vera), some are dry (such as nettle), some are cold (such as mints), and some are hot (such as cayenne). As such, grouping them in some way to best align the herbal energetics with the person's energetics was necessary for proper treatment.

In many other traditional systems of medicine, there is a similar categorization. TCM divides people into nine constitutions or body types. In the Western Vitalist tradition that Danielle was trained in, there are four constitutions or body types. People fall into one of four constitutions, connected to the elements of air, water, fire, and earth. These have associated temperatures and moistures to them. Air is hot and wet; water is cold and wet; fire is hot and dry, and earth is cold and dry.

If this sounds a bit heady, let's break it down. Every person is prone to be a bit more moist or dry (literally and figuratively). This is somewhat assigned at birth, but can also be affected by the foods you are eating or the climate you are living in. For example, if you live by the ocean, you may have a moister constitution than someone who lives in the mountains at several thousand feet of elevation where the climate is naturally dry. The moisture of your body can be recognized by your skin, digestion, and general tissue state. The expression of these systems lets you know if you are overly boggy or excessively dried out.

Additionally, we all fall on the temperature spectrum of hot or dry. This can also be influenced by lifestyle factors such as environment, exercise, and diet. Yet temperature and moisture are also somewhat assigned at birth. Even if siblings live in the same place, are fed the same diet, drink the same water, and engage in the same activities, one may be more fiery and outgoing while the other may be shier and quieter.

Let us go through a brief example. Two people present with the exact same symptom profile: they are experiencing the same digestive complaints. One person has a hot and dry constitution (fire, pitta). The other has a moist and cold constitution (water, earth, kapha).

Even though ginger is a common medicine for stomach upset, we must recognize that it is a hot and dry root. If it is ingested by an already hot and dry body, it may push the person's system farther over the edge, perhaps making their symptoms worse.

However, if that same ginger is given to the moist and cold body, it may bring about great healing. Therefore, we must preface that while the Adaptogens listed in this book are categorized in a way more familiar to our modern-day usage and understanding, it is critical to understand both your personal and natural medicine energetics to truly choose the right natural medicine for your needs at varying times.

Understanding which body type, constitution, temperament, or dosha you are is fundamental to using whole, natural medicines, including Adaptogens. Check out the following chart to help you discover your unique constitution.

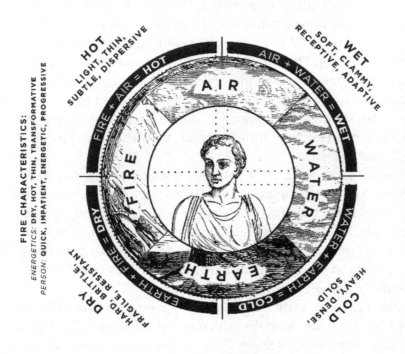

AIR CHARACTERISTICS:
ENERGETICS: WET, HOT, THIN, SUBTLE, MUTABLE
PERSON: ASPIRING, IDEALISTIC, EASILY DISTRACTED

EARTH CHARACTERISTICS:
ENERGETICS: DRY, COLD, HEAVY, DENSE, COMPACT
PERSON: DILIGENT, HONEST, STEADFAST, GROUNDED

We encourage you to learn about your own body type to choose the best allies and natural medicines for your unique needs. There are also amazing natural practitioners that can help guide you to the right options for your body.

ADAPTOGENS' EMERGENCE IN MODERN TIMES

Once upon a time in a land far, far away—specifically, the U.S.S.R. (modern-day Russia) 1940—top Soviet scientist and military doctor Nikolai Lazarev, with his team of Russian scientists, went on a mission to find the most powerful substances on the planet to fight stress, prevent or reduce illness, strengthen the body and mind, and foster a strong and resilient population. Dr. Lazarev was particularly interested in the potential of traditional plant medicines to help soldiers with strength and stamina. One of his team's first studies in the 1950s illuminated the powerful effects of Ginseng. This broke new ground and paved the way for them to continue to find similar species that "are medicinal substances causing the state of nonspecifically increased resistance" against stress.[1] Their team searched the globe and after years of research, landed on a group of natural medicines they decided to call *Adaptogens*.

The word comes from the Latin word *adaptare*, meaning to fit or adjust. The first definition from Dr. Lazarev in 1947 was "an agent that allows your body to counter adverse physical, chemical, or biological stressors by raising nonspecific resistance toward such stress, thus allowing the organism to 'adapt' to the stressful circumstances."[2] This definition is still the foundation for the modern-day understanding of Adaptogens.

After Lazarev's early definition of Adaptogens was coined, one of his students, long-time friends, and mentees, Dr. Israel Brekhman, continued to study these rare herbs and fungi for the next 50 years. He was fascinated by their ability to withstand stressors in nature, such as surviving ice ages and living under extreme environmental conditions. He proposed that these qualities could help the human body adapt and deal with similar stressors. (Hence the name, *adapt*-ogens. They give our bodies the tools to better adapt to whatever stressors life throws our way.)

Dr. Brekhman expanded his team and gathered around 1,200 physicians and biologists to investigate these species. They went on to conduct over 3,000 studies on the initial group of Adaptogenic flora and fungi. These studies and clinical trials were the first scientific evidence of the profound immune and stress-protective properties of these species. The research further proved that they are nontoxic, improve physical and mental performance, aid in stress management, and have an overall benefit to balance the systems of your body.

For the past several decades, these species have undergone gold standard (randomized, double-blind, and placebo-controlled) clinical trials to see if their ancient use could be confirmed by modern science. It turns out, while research continues to be conducted, the complexity of these species, the ability for them to interact with multiple systems of the body, and to bring about profound healing benefits has been seen through the lens of both history and science. This intersection—a deep history of use with generations of stories and trials combined with modern research—makes Adaptogens an incredibly intriguing asset to our modern times.

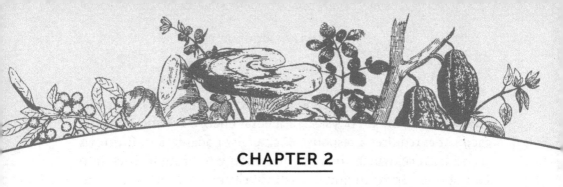

CHAPTER 2

ADAPTOGENS FOR WHOLE-BODY HEALTH

Now that you know about the traditional systems Adaptogens came from as well as the story that brought them to the Western eye, let's marry the old and the new. This context is our suggested way of viewing Adaptogens to reap the most benefits. It's a combination of the traditional views married with the science of modern-day thought; a vision of bringing key concepts from both the old (Ayurveda and TCM) and the new (Western medicine). This is a fresh lens for you to hold through the remainder of the book (and ideally, the remainder of your life with Adaptogens!).

Think of your body as an ecosystem. One that is constantly calibrating, in a rhythmic dance, to keep the thousands of operations constantly happening in your body functioning optimally. There is a threshold where we feel our best. It includes a specific range of blood sugar levels, temperature, amount of carbon dioxide in our lungs, and more. Keeping these systems in balance means our immune systems can effectively protect us against invaders, our minds can fire neurons optimally enough to grow and expand, and we can fall asleep with ease, essentially living in a state of health and vitality. The most common way to throw off this beautiful balance is stress.

Stress is defined as a forcibly exerted pressure that causes distress and demand on physical or mental energy. Essentially, it is a factor that requires a response of change or adaptation. It throws us off balance, which then requires energy to bring us back into equilibrium. Stress in and of itself isn't bad; it's a brilliant evolutionary response.

Our stress response goes way back. As humans, the earliest stressors we encountered were threats to our survival. A prime example of early evolutionary stress is an animal coming to attack us. In this acute situation, stress is required to survive. Our bodies enter a state of fight, flight, freeze, or fawn. Our adrenal glands immediately flood our bloodstream with hormones like cortisol and adrenaline. These give us the energy needed to fight off the animal about to attack us or to run for our life. These hormones trigger systemic bodily responses: increased blood pressure, more rapid breathing, a release of sugar into the bloodstream for quick energy, and more. In this moment of acute stress, all energy is diverted to survival.

In the moments right before an animal attack, do you think your body is giving you signals about whether you are hungry, tired, or horny? Of course not! All other systems go on "airplane mode." Digestion, immune function, sex drive, and other secondary physiological functions not critical to immediate survival are suppressed. They take the back seat so that all your energy is available to respond to the acute perceived threat. This stress response has enabled us, as humans, to survive many obstacles over the course of our existence.

The problem arises when stress becomes chronic. Unfortunately, in today's world, we are no longer experiencing this systemic, body-wide state of stress strictly in moments of acute survival. Even worse, when the stressor does occur, we are not fighting or running, burning off all those stress hormones and allowing our bodies to then return to a state of balance.

Instead, stressors occur daily, if not every few minutes or hour. Listening to the news—boom! Stress response. Driving to work, someone cuts you off—boom! Stress response. Get to work, boss sends an angry e-mail—boom! Stress response. It's on and on and on. Then we sit in our cars or at our offices or in front of our TVs with all these powerful stress hormones circulating in our system. It's no wonder we get headaches, gain weight, have low energy, have difficulty falling asleep, and the many other common symptoms of today.

Our bodies, on a physiological level, think they're in survival mode—nearly all the time. The messages about when we are hungry, tired, horny, and other basic biological functions of being a human are literally turned off. It's only when we can get out of this acute state of stress that other systems can turn on again. It's like a pin pressing on a very specific part of your body. When it's pressing in, all you can feel and notice is that specific point. When the pin is released, the energy is diverted back all over your body where it's meant to be.

The state of the world has conditioned us to be constantly awaiting the next stressor. Pins on pins. Physiologically, our bloodstream is repeatedly flooded with stress hormones to keep us on high alert. Continued high levels of stress hormones lead to physical and mental exhaustion. Not to stress you out, but over time, this leads to psychological and physical damage.

But knowing that we can't quite avoid all the stressors of daily life, how do we support our bodies in dealing with all this stress? We believe that the single most powerful, safe, and natural way to combat this stress cycle is with Adaptogens.

SCIENCE OF HOW ADAPTOGENS
WORK IN OUR BODIES

What does normalizing really mean? Let us walk you through each of the main systems of your body so you can understand how Adaptogens help bring balance to the immune and gastrointestinal systems, neurological and endocrinal systems, and circulatory and respiratory systems.

Adaptogens affect all systems of your body. Many have a strong influence on the endocrine, nervous, and immune systems, but different systems in your body are affected more strongly than others by certain Adaptogens. We'll go into depth about the neuroendocrine association with Adaptogens (particularly Reishi and Ashwagandha), as well as the immune system (where most functional mushrooms shine). We'll then go through the other systems of your body explaining how Adaptogens interact, balance, and replenish each of these areas of your body.

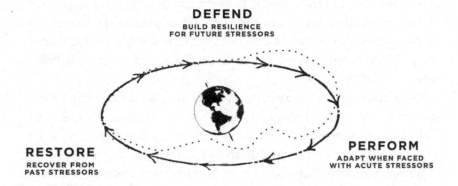

DEFEND
BUILD RESILIENCE
FOR FUTURE STRESSORS

RESTORE
RECOVER FROM
PAST STRESSORS

PERFORM
ADAPT WHEN FACED
WITH ACUTE STRESSORS

Defend: **Immune System + Digestive System:** These systems are interconnected, as about 70 percent of immune cells are located in the gut (microbiome). The health of the gut is therefore intricately related to the strength of the body's immune system. Adaptogens greatly support these systems via their immunomodulating activity. We like to think of immunomodulation as cruise control for the immune system. If the immune system is underactive—in times of stress or cold and flu season—an immunomodulator can *stimulate* immune cell activity. If the immune system is overactive—as in autoimmune conditions—an immunomodulator can also *down-regulate* immune activity. All functional mushrooms mentioned in this book are immunomodulators. There are several plant Adaptogens that also help to balance and strengthen the immune system.

When it comes to the digestive system, there are few areas that have more active research than gut health. We are starting to understand that the microbiome is not only relevant to digestion itself, but is an integral component of immunity, mood, sleep, and even skin health. There are more microorganisms residing in our gut than there are human cells in our body, and the balance of these organisms determines the expression of health. Everything we eat is feeding either the good or bad organisms in our gut. Luckily, Adaptogens' complex phytochemical profiles replenish the gut with ample amounts of vitamins, minerals, amino acids, and even prebiotics to support a thriving gut ecosystem.

In brief, the immune support and gut health Adaptogens help prepare you to defend against modern-day stressors.

Perform: **Circulatory (Cardiovascular) + Respiratory System:** The Circulatory system includes the heart, blood vessels (including veins, arteries, and capillaries), and blood. The lymphatic system is often considered a supplementary system to the circulatory system. The main job of this system is to send sufficient supplies of blood (oxygen and nutrients) to all tissues, organs, muscles, and bones in your body. This transportation system nourishes cells, removes metabolic waste, and destroys pathogens that may be present within the bloodstream.

It is also intricately connected to the reproductive system, as circulation is a key component to libido. As you'll later learn, certain Adaptogens like Eleuthero and Ginseng have a particular affinity for stimulating the circulatory system. Proper blood flow to sexual organs is essential for arousal and pleasure. Libido supportive Adaptogens often affect the circulatory system, by increasing blood flow and delivering nutrient-rich blood to the sexual organs. This is how they help increase performance.

Closely related to the circulatory system is the respiratory system. This system regulates the exchange of air (oxygen and carbon dioxide) in and out of your body. While commonly thought of as involuntary, it is one of the most unique and fascinating systems of your body. It can operate without thought or intention but can also be highly manipulated with mindful intent. The control of this system has a systemic effect on your body.

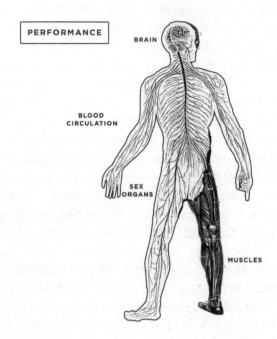

Fascinating ancient research combined with newer exper-imental trials are revealing just how powerful this system can be for whole-body health. Without Adaptogens, when a stressor occurs, one of its autonomic responses is to increase the heart rate which increases breathing. Breathing too fast leads to hyperven-tilation. The faster you breathe, the more oxygen your body takes in. This prepares your body for "fight or flight."

When the amount of air your body is receiving and releasing changes, the entire chemistry of your body shifts. Adaptogens, by reducing the intensity of the reaction to a stressor, reduce the bodily response of increased heart rate and rapid breathing. As a result, there is a steadying of the breath and respiratory system. This allows your body to conserve energy, stay calm, and approach the stressor from a place of stability. It also enables the energy that would have been locked up in breathing and increased heart rate to be diverted to other organs of your body, like the brain and the sexual organs.

We believe that the way Adaptogens affect this system may be a key reason for their stress-supportive and whole-body protective effects. To put the importance of this system in context, Tero likes to remind us that a person can survive weeks without food, days without water, but only minutes without breath. Control of these systems, therefore, is essential to maintenance and regulation of every other system in your body.

The circulatory and respiratory Adaptogens are for when you need to perform against the acute stressors you are facing.

Restore: **Neuroendocrine System (NES):** This is the system that is controlled by neurotransmitters and hormone-chemical messengers found throughout your body. It is the connection between the nervous system and the endocrinal or hormonal system. This system includes the central components of the hypothalamus, pituitary, and adrenal glands, or the hypothalamic–pituitary–adrenal (HPA) axis, and monitors hormone production, including regulating stress.

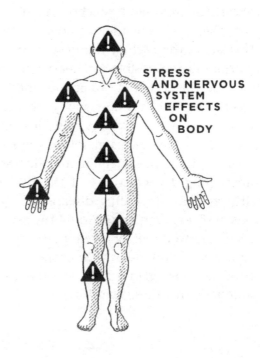

STRESS AND NERVOUS SYSTEM EFFECTS ON BODY

One of the fundamental ways Adaptogens are thought to support stress and balance in your body is via the HPA axis. It is occasionally referred to as the HPAT, which includes T for "thyroid," but we'll refer to it as the HPA here.

The *hypothalamus* is a small yet crucial part of the brain. It acts as the control center for several autonomic functions, including sleep, growth, appetite, and body temperature. It links the nervous system to the endocrine system via the *pituitary gland*, a pea-sized gland in the brain often called the "master gland." Small but mighty, it is located at the base of the brain behind the bridge of the nose and produces hormones that control several important functions in your body. It's responsible for releasing adrenocorticotropic hormone into the blood, which signals the adrenal cortex to secrete corticoids and signals the adrenal medulla to release norepinephrine. In conjunction with the hypothalamus, the pituitary gland is responsible for the release of many hormones including cortisol (the stress hormone). Next comes the *adrenals*, the two glands that sit above the kidneys in the back. They are responsible for the release of hormones that enable the body to respond to stress (like corticosteroids and catecholamines).

The last gland occasionally included in this system is the *thyroid*. This sits at the back of the neck near the windpipe and controls hormones responsible for heart rate, temperature, and metabolism. Together, the HPA can be thought of as the endocrine energy director that controls how your body reacts to stress on a physiological level. When stressors arise, it is mediated through the HPA axis. This system helps maintain stress-related hormones to keep the heart, immune system, metabolic system, and nervous system functioning. Hyperactivity of the HPA axis is central to most health problems, including disease and aging. When your body is constantly exposed to stressors—the news, traffic, strained relationships, overworking, or even pesticides, herbicides, and plastics—it negatively interferes with proper HPA functioning. All these stressors tax these glands and in turn weaken the many systems in your body that these glands regulate.

Let's look at what happens when your body is under chronic stress and the HPA is taxed. The three main consequences of HPA disruption are immune suppression, brain impairment, and aging. The adrenals secrete large amounts of vitamin C and vitamin B5 when under stress. Vitamin C is a crucial component of a healthy immune system (along with a laundry list of other important benefits in your body). Vitamin B5 is part of your body's cellular energy supply. With the flooding of these vitamins, the immune system becomes weakened and susceptible to antigens.

Adaptogens can spare the adrenal glands from losing vitamin C, preventing the immune system from taking too deep of a toll from the stress. The brain is also affected by prolonged stress hormones. Elevated levels of cortisol and glucocorticoids have been linked to memory impairment.[1] Finally, when the glands of the HPA are overtaxed, organ systems begin to deteriorate. With constant taxing, they are forced to try and reestablish balance repeatedly. Over time, this leads to hyperactivation of the HPA and too much cortisol.

Excess cortisol promotes catabolism or breaking down and atrophy of muscle, organ tissues, and even bone density. This is where Adaptogens can be directly and physiologically supportive and protective to aging, immunity, brain health, and more. Adaptogens give our bodies the tools to respond and recover from stress more efficiently, preventing the downward spiral and exhaustion of the HPA. They can mitigate the hormone imbalances that occur from stress and aging. Their antioxidants, polysaccharides, triterpenes, and range of other compounds help to keep your body feeling youthful and balanced.

The neuroendocrine system Adaptogens are for when you need to restore and replenish your system from the many stressors of daily life.

While the Defend, Perform, and Restore categorization system is meant to make it easier to understand the main systems of your body that Adaptogens interact with, always remember that your body is an ecosystem where everything affects everything else.

There are 11 systems in your body in total. Adaptogens interact with the six systems above (nervous, endocrine, immune, digestive, cardiovascular, and respiratory), as well as the other five systems inadvertently (skeletal, reproductive, muscular, urinary, and integumentary). Adaptogens are nonspecific, so the way they affect the systems of your body often happens in a cascade reaction. One change affects everything downstream. For example, a change in breath rate affects the chemistry of the blood, which affects the cardiovascular system, changing the alertness of the brain, blocking blood flow to the sexual organs, and thus affecting libido, and so on.

LIST OF BODY SYSTEMS

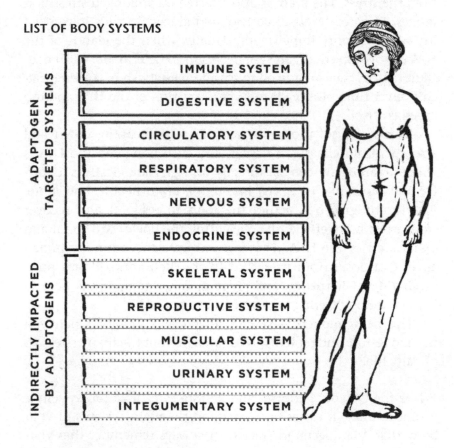

ADAPTOGEN TARGETED SYSTEMS

- IMMUNE SYSTEM
- DIGESTIVE SYSTEM
- CIRCULATORY SYSTEM
- RESPIRATORY SYSTEM
- NERVOUS SYSTEM
- ENDOCRINE SYSTEM

INDIRECTLY IMPACTED BY ADAPTOGENS

- SKELETAL SYSTEM
- REPRODUCTIVE SYSTEM
- MUSCULAR SYSTEM
- URINARY SYSTEM
- INTEGUMENTARY SYSTEM

UNDERSTANDING THE SCIENCE
THROUGH KEY COMPOUNDS

At this point, you know that when it comes to Adaptogens, the whole is greater than the sum of its parts. Essentially, there is more benefit when using a whole plant or mushroom, as opposed to an isolated compound from that species. That said, modern science needs to pick apart and name compounds to assess exactly how they impact your body. Since this book is a combination of both traditional wisdom and modern scientific research, we must break down a few of the categories of compounds that are found in many Adaptogens.

When analyzing a clinical trial that aims to prove the medicinal or functional benefits of a plant or mushroom, specific compounds are traced to understand how they interact with certain parts of our bodies to create beneficial results. Many of these compounds are known as phytochemicals, "phyto" meaning "plant," and "chemicals" being the tiny entities (atoms) that make up the structure of say minerals (like magnesium) or sugars (polysaccharides). These are the key phytochemicals in Adaptogens:

Saponins: Saponins come from the Latin word for soap, *sapo*. They have soap-like qualities and can produce foam when mixed with water. Some original saponin-containing plants were used as the first natural soaps.

Yet beyond utility, they have incredible health benefits. Their soap-like effect allows them to bind to fat-soluble molecules and bile acids in your body's gastrointestinal tract. They help eliminate the toxins (and bad cholesterol) and prevent them from getting reabsorbed by your body. A catchy way to remember them is the phytochemicals that "wash away" unwanted toxins from your body (just like soap externally).

Additionally, saponins support immune health through their antimicrobial, antifungal, antiparasitic, and insecticidal properties.[2,3] Plants depend on saponins to fight against these various pathogens in nature. Lucky for us, when we consume plant saponins, we get similar protective benefits. Some famous saponins include ginsenosides from Ginseng and gypenosides from Gynostemma.

Polysaccharides: Polysaccharides are long sugar chains, most famous for their immune system support. In Latin, "poly" means "many," and saccharides are sugars. These molecular chains are found in the rigid cell walls of mushrooms as well as some Adaptogenic plants including Ginseng, Goji, Astragalus, and Eleuthero. Many cells that are part of your body's immune system, including macrophages, NK cells, dendritic cells, neutrophils, and monocytes, have specific receptors for polysaccharides.

The most common polysaccharides found in functional mushrooms are 1,3 and 1,6 beta-D-glucans. Polysaccharides are the compounds responsible for modulating immune cells. They are antibacterial and antiviral, and can stimulate or suppress immune activity as needed. They can be found in plants other than Adaptogens (like oats and algae), but in functional mushrooms there is the greatest variety.

Newer research also points to beta-glucans' benefit to gut health.[4] They act as prebiotics, essential components of a healthy microbiome. Prebiotics are like food for probiotics (good bacteria in your gut). They can increase the number of diverse healthy bacteria in the gut, which can also improve the immune system and whole-body health.

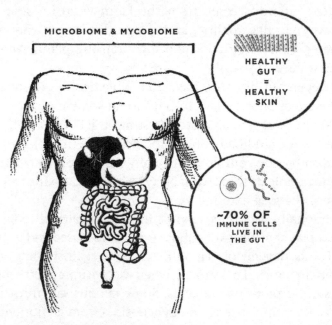

MICROBIOME & MYCOBIOME

HEALTHY
GUT
=
HEALTHY
SKIN

~70% OF
IMMUNE CELLS
LIVE IN
THE GUT

Triterpenes: Triterpenes are a specific type of terpenes. Terpenes are found in all flora and fungi. We like to think of them in layman's terms like nature's oils. They are often responsible for the aroma of nature, such as the terpene linalool, an essential oil of lavender, or cineol (sometimes called eucalyptol) that gives tea tree its strong scent. As some of the oldest medicines in nature, terpenes have been used for millennia, such as when resins of pine and eucalyptus are inhaled to cure a cold. The word "terpene" was coined from "turpentine," which came from the resin of pine trees. It was traditionally used as an antiseptic for wound cleaning, and later the "turp" prefix was left out, creating the term "terpene."

Plants and mushrooms use terpenes as part of their defense systems. Triterpenes have three terpene units and a slightly more complex molecular structure. There are over 5,000 triterpenes in nature, many found in functional mushrooms. Triterpenes have been studied for their numerous biological activities including anti-tumor, anti-inflammatory, hepatoprotective, immunomodulating, antimicrobial, antibacterial, anti-hepatitis, antioxidant, hypoglycemic, anti-malarial, and anti-HIV properties.[5] These are the second most abundant metabolites (group of compounds) in functional mushrooms, just behind polysaccharides.

Primarily found in the fruiting bodies of fungi, triterpenes are responsible for the bitter taste of real mushroom extracts. Triterpenes are particularly good at killing bacteria and viruses. They exert an anti-inflammatory effect, which prevents excess inflammation without preventing white blood cells from doing their job. This unique ability to stimulate your body's natural immune defenses, without pushing too far, is where triterpenes differ from many other natural immune remedies. Examples include ganoderic acids from Reishi mushroom and betulinic acid from Chaga. Triterpenes are also found in Ginseng, Astragalus, Eleuthero, and Tulsi.

Antioxidants: These are so important to overall health, longevity, and foundational wellness that they are present in nearly every Adaptogen we discuss. Antioxidants are mostly found in the colorful pigments in flora or fungi. The dark black pigments that give Chaga mushroom its color, the bright red of Schisandra berries or

Acerola cherries, and even certain vitamins (like A, C, and E) act as antioxidants. They act as scavengers, looking for "free radicals."

Free radicals are dangerous, unbound molecules that attack and steal electrons from other molecules. Once a molecule has been attacked and stolen from (this is all on an atomic level), it becomes a free radical itself. Essentially, a domino effect quickly occurs.

If your body doesn't have a sufficient supply of antioxidants to bind to these free radicals and stop the cascade, oxidative damage begins to occur. Oxidative stress or damage has been linked to several conditions that negatively affect the brain, heart, lungs and can even lead to cancers.[6] Unfortunately, free radicals are unavoidable.

Some normally arise from daily activities like metabolism, exercise, and aging. Others come from environmental factors such as radiation, pollution, smoke, herbicides, pesticides, and heavy metals. Antioxidants are "free radical scavengers." They neutralize, prevent, and repair the damage done by free radicals.

Phenols: This is the largest category of phytochemicals. The three most important phenols for dietary purposes are flavonoids, phenolic acids, and polyphenols.

Flavonoids are a powerful group of plant metabolites that have shown anti-inflammatory, antioxidant, anti-mutagenic, anti-aging, and even anticancer activity.[7] There are over 4,000 subtypes of flavonoids. The most common types with medicinal benefits are anthocyanins (found in Acerola), flavanols (found in Cacao), and isoflavones (found in Astragalus).

Phenolic acids are most noteworthy for their antioxidant activity. They are also antimicrobial, anticancer, anti-inflammatory, and anti-mutagenic.[8] Phenolic acids are found in Acerola, Moringa, Mucuna, and Turkey Tail mushrooms.

Lastly, *polyphenols* can be thought of as antioxidants that act like Adaptogens to plants. They help plants tolerate various stressors and are found in Turmeric, Mucuna, Cacao, Turkey Tail, and Acerola. Each subgroup of phenols plays an incredibly important role in protecting your body from stress, toxins, and chronic inflammation.

These natural compounds are some of the foundational constitu-ents in Adaptogens that give them their premier status.

Adaptogens also contain other famous compounds such as vitamins, minerals, alkaloids, and healthy lipids, but they are more specific to individual species. This is also a good opportu-nity to remember that what is so unique about whole plant and mushroom medicine (as opposed to Western pharmaceuticals, which are composed of isolated compounds often originating from the natural environment) is that there are always multiple compounds working in concert to create an effect in your body.

When science tries to isolate a compound, the results may fall short because it may not be any isolated compound that results in the benefit but rather the combination of how they work together. Adaptogens are whole plants and mushrooms that, when used properly, can have profound benefits to raising baseline vitality.

PART II

THE
21
ESSENTIAL
ADAPTOGENS

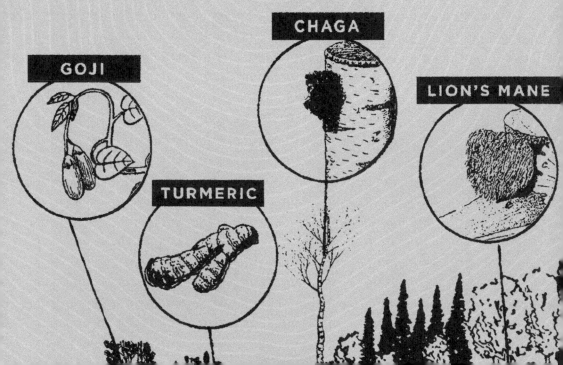

GOJI

CHAGA

LION'S MANE

TURMERIC

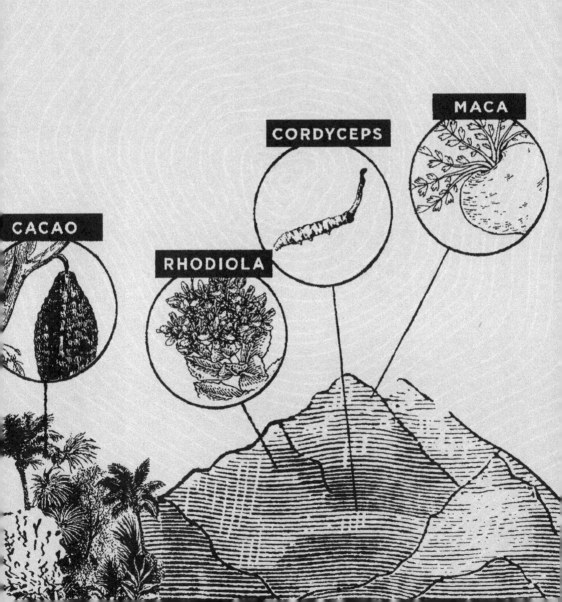

W e've come to the exciting part of this book: the Adaptogen profiles. Each profile begins with a fun fact box. Then, we'll dive deeper into each Adaptogen's full potential.

Full legal name: The Latin name of each species and its taxonomic family. This is important because common names or nicknames differ across the world. Every language has a different name for a species, or sometimes even many names. The Latin name, however, doesn't change around the world or based on what language you speak. Just like your full legal name, it stays with you no matter where you travel.

Nicknames: Common names. These are shorthand names or names in different languages. Depending on who you are talking to or what ancient text you are reading, you may come across some of these names. It's another tool to know what species you are getting acquainted with.

Power hub: The part of the plant or mushroom that is used medicinally. This is the area that contains the most benefits for health.

Home: The place(s) of origin where the Adaptogen is found in nature.

Energetics: The temperature (hot, cold, neutral) and moisture (moist, dry, neutral) of the Adaptogen. Use this information to help you to find the Adaptogen that will best align with your unique constitution.

Helpful with: The top three benefits of the Adaptogen, which will be elaborated on later in the profile.

Comes with: The key constituents or phytochemicals found in this Adaptogen. They're important to call out for two reasons. First, they will help you understand the clinical trials and modern research associated with the Adaptogen. Second, you can begin to familiarize yourself with its compounds and benefits.

Common uses: The occasions and situations that the Adaptogen is particularly helpful with.

Best friends: Other ingredients that the Adaptogen has synergistic effects with. Consider using any combination of the Adaptogen with one or a few of these ingredients to enhance its effect.

Each fact box is followed by a quick introduction on that Adaptogen's history (the ancient wisdom, long history of use in cultures around the world, and thus time-tested functionality of these ingredients); an in-depth analysis of its key benefits; instructions for preparing, sourcing, and dosing; and practical suggestions for how to use it. We've purposely included scientific studies in the "helpful with" sections to illustrate their powers through modern research. This book is meant to be a perennial guide to Adaptogens. We encourage reading through the ingredient profiles, experimenting with the Adaptogen in your own life, and then exploring the referenced studies (all of which can be found at the end of the book) to keep your journey with Adaptogens well rounded and continually evolving.

HOW TO USE THE CATEGORIES: DEFEND, PERFORM, RESTORE

Much like TCM and Ayurveda, we created a categorization system that we hope will make it easy for you to navigate this book and use the Adaptogens. Like the ancient classification systems, our classification system addresses the underlying cause of your issue or ailment and aims to raise your Qi, or vital energy, for healing. At the same time, it integrates the modern understanding of choosing a course of action or treatment based on its benefits.

Similarly, each Adaptogen profile shares the energetics of each Adaptogen but also the main benefits it may be used for. This allows you to begin to understand the Adaptogens based on where they are from, their moisture and temperature level, and their top benefits.

Danielle often tells her clients, the medicine doesn't work if you don't take it. What this means is, practicality is everything. No matter how incredible an Adaptogen might be for you, if it tastes horrible, is completely outside of your routine, or simply is offered in a form that is unfamiliar to you, the chances are, you won't take it. And the thing with Adaptogens is they must be taken not once, but consistently, to truly reap the benefits. Therefore, the first step to receiving the benefits from these incredible species is for you to understand why and how to use them. To do that, we need to share this information in a way that addresses where most people need support: Defend, Perform, and Restore.

Defend: Immune Support and Skin Protection

Are you trying to **Defend** your body from viruses and chronic sniffles? What about ditching seasonal allergies for good? Or to finally achieve that dewy glow that no amount of fancy skin products seems to do the trick with? Or are you interested in beauty practices to prevent your skin—your largest organ—from potential damage before it happens?

In the Defend section, you will find three Adaptogens known for *Immunity* (Chaga, Eleuthero, and Turkey Tail) and four Adaptogens acclaimed for their *Beauty and Skin* benefits (Turmeric, Goji, Schisandra, and Acerola).

Perform: Physically or Mentally

Do you need more physical energy to power through the day? Are you seeking more endurance in your physical activity or simply performing day-to-day functions? Are you looking for more vitality in the bedroom? Are you ready to finally say good-bye to brain fog?

In this section, you'll find three powerful clean energy species (Ginseng, Cordyceps, and Maca). Since more energy is not always better, better energy is better, the Perform section also includes four amazing Adaptogens for *Brain and Focus* (Lion's Mane, Mucuna, Gotu Kola, and Rhodiola). These seven Adaptogens can help your body perform when needed, without hurting the restoration phase which will follow after a busy spurt.

Restore: Stress Support, Rest, and Mood

Do you need deep relaxation? Are you having trouble falling or staying asleep? Are you often wired, needing a dose of calm to enhance your mood? Or are you trying to biohack yourself to live 100-plus years full of life?

Sometimes you need help with *Stress and Mood* before anything else. Here we have three of our absolute favorite allies (Ashwagandha, Reishi, and Tulsi) for daily recovery and stress support. Since we're all about long-term health, we also unpack four amazing Adaptogens for *Longevity and Well-Being* (Cacao, Gynostemma, Moringa, and Astragalus). These seven Adaptogens round out the routine, helping to nourish and restore your body.

Keep in mind that while Adaptogens are categorized in this book in Defend, Perform, and Restore categories, this is not *all* these species are good for. As you'll soon learn, part of what makes Adaptogens so unique is their multifaceted approach to supporting your body. Categorizing highlights their *main* benefits for the beginning of your Adaptogenic journey. As you become more familiar with them, stay open to discovering even more benefits than what meets the page.

GETTING THE MOST OUT OF THE ADAPTOGENS

You can read the following 21 Adaptogen profiles straight through or you can jump to the Adaptogens you're most interested in first. If you're still wondering which Adaptogen is right for you, review the following:

- Profiles for the Defend, Perform, and Restore categories in this chapter
- "Helpful with" and "Comes with" sections in the fact boxes
- Energetics section in the fact boxes (after determining your body's energetic constitution through the chart on p. 11)

Once you see something that calls to your needs or body type, read on for a deeper understanding of the Adaptogen.

Now the long-awaited time has finally come. It is time to meet the 21 Adaptogens to start your journey with the most powerful, nutrient-dense, and revered species on the planet!

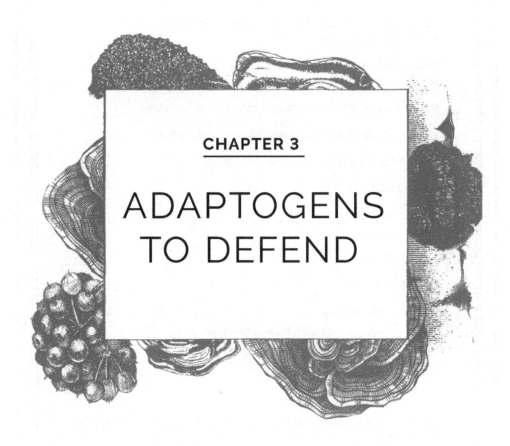

CHAPTER 3

ADAPTOGENS TO DEFEND

FOR IMMUNITY AND PROTECTION

CHAGA

Full legal name: *Inonotus obliquus,* from the fungi "crust" family, *Hymenochaetaceae* (the rotters)

Nicknames: King of mushrooms, clinker polypore, cancer fungus. Hates being called a sclerotium.

Power hub: Sterile conk growing outside the birch tree

Home: Siberia, Scandinavia, and Northeast America

Energetics: Neutral temperature, slightly dry

Helpful with:

1. Immunity
2. Longevity
3. Beauty

Comes with:

- Antioxidants
- Triterpenoids: Betulin and betulinic acid
- SOD (superoxide dismutase)
- Melanin
- Polysaccharides

Common uses: Early mornings or keeping you going during long winter days

Best friends: Eleuthero, coffee, rose hips, cinnamon, and elderberry

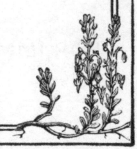

A BRIEF HISTORY: From a Fire Starter to a Cancer Aid to a Coffee Alternative

Chaga is known as the "king of mushrooms." Its uses over time have been diverse, and Chaga may take the win for the strangest uses of all Adaptogens. It's been used as utility or medicine in every place it grows (mostly northern, colder climates). In Canada, native Cree healers used it as incense and as tinder for fires. In Siberia, Khanty healers would use it for digestive issues. In China, it is burned as moxibustion (an ancient practice of burning herbs over acupressure points to treat ailments). And in Siberia, women bathe in Chaga tea as a cleansing ritual while menstruating. Additional traditional uses include blood purification, pain relief, cancer cure, and immune support.

One of our favorite Chaga stories relates to Tero's not-too-distant relatives. In Finland, where Tero was born and raised, people drink more coffee per capita than any other place in the world. The average is about five to six cups per day! During coffee rations in WWII, Finns couldn't get enough coffee beans, so they brewed Chaga instead. When brewed, Chaga is a jet-black color with an earthy flavor that resembles coffee. It was a hit! It's now added into coffee in upscale restaurants and trendy food trucks to add more function to coffee. Its remarkable antioxidant profile, immune benefits, and ease of use make it a no-brainer for daily consumption.

HELPFUL WITH IMMUNITY

Chaga is best known for its immune support, and for good reason. In 1966, Russian author and Nobel laureate Aleksandr Solzhenitsyn wrote in his book *The Cancer Ward* that Chaga cured his cancerous tumor. This started the conversation in the West around the potential for Chaga to support immunity. Today, Chaga is known for its antitumor and anticancer activity. In a 2016 study from Japan, rats with cancerous tumors were given six milligrams per kilogram of their weight per day of a Chaga decoction. After three weeks, their tumors were reduced in size by 60 percent. The study concluded that Chaga extract suppresses cancer by promoting energy metabolism.[1] It's also quite antiviral, key to fighting off viral disease, including herpes simplex virus (HSV) and human immunodeficiency virus (HIV).[2,3] Its antiviral activity has even been studied for its potential effectiveness against SARS-CoV-2,[4] but more research is needed.

The methods of action in which Chaga supports the immune system are varied. Some research shows it induces apoptosis (cell death) of cancer cells.[5] Other research points to its abundant antioxidants, which help combat the negative side effects of disease.[6] Additionally, its polysaccharides modulate the immune system. Like many whole substances found in nature, there are a multitude of compounds working together to give Chaga its protective effects on the immune system.[7,8] Chaga's trifecta of immune compounds (beta glucans, antioxidants, and triterpenes) make it a great choice to use alongside conventional immune support.

HELPFUL FOR LONGEVITY

As we age, our body breaks down, both physically and mentally. On a cellular level, aging is literally cell death or atrophy. Stress is a leading cause of cellular atrophy. We don't mean just stress over a to-do list, the news, kids, and work. A 2019 study found that the polysaccharides from Chaga known as *Inonotus obliquus* polysaccharides (IOPS) modulated oxidative stress and slowed down mitochondrial apoptosis. This means the mitochondria stayed alive longer, despite stressors. It also shows that with the help of IOPS, stress can be recovered from without leading to cell death.[9,10] Other research confirms Chaga can "prevent the aging process by attenuating oxidative stress."[11]

Another inevitable effect of aging is slowing down. Mental and physical exhaustion cause the body to move at a slower pace. Chaga has the potential to postpone physical fatigue and improve mental fatigue.[12] A 14-day study showed that Chaga extended the swimming time of mice with no toxic effects on any organs, confirming its anti-fatigue potential.[13] The longer the body takes to break down and slow down, the longer we live.

HELPFUL FOR BEAUTY

Chaga contains an astonishing number of antioxidants that are particularly beneficial for skin health and beauty. First, it is one of the most abundant food sources of melanin, which is the dark pigment responsible for the color of human skin, hair, and eyes. Melanin's job is to protect the body, specifically the skin, from the negative effects of oxidative stress, such as sun damage. Think of Chaga like an anti-aging serum that works from the inside out. Melanin is also a potent antioxidant with one of the highest ORAC (oxygen radical absorbance capacity) scores. In fact, Chaga has about 1,300 times the number of antioxidants as blueberries! Chaga also contains betulinic acid, an antibacterial, antiviral, and anti-inflammatory compound that protects the skin against all sorts of trouble, including inhibiting the growth of melanoma (skin cancer) cells.[14]

Chaga's antioxidants have been used to support skin health both topically and internally for hundreds of years. Chaga contains SOD (superoxide dismutase), an enzyme naturally present in all human cells. Its role is to break down superoxide radicals, which can be damaging to your body's cells. In this way, it provides cellular defense to protect cells from becoming mutated or damaged. SOD is mostly used as an anti-aging supplement.

Chaga has even been shown to help psoriasis, a skin disease thought to have no cure. Psoriasis causes the skin to break out in red, itchy patches, where the skin may crack, burn, or scale off. Over time, it can affect the joints and cause chronic pain and discomfort. The only medications on the market act as bandages, temporarily easing symptoms. Yet a Russian study that tested 50 patients with psoriasis found that with consistent internal and external use of Chaga extract, 14 patients were completely cured. The others had significant improvements in symptoms, all without any negative side effects.[15]

PREPARATION, SOURCING, AND DOSAGE

When sourcing Chaga, the most important thing to look for is wild harvested. Real Chaga must be harvested out in nature, where it primarily grows on birch trees. Some of Chaga's key compounds like betulinic acid come from the bark of the birch tree. Avoid lab grown Chaga "mushroom" mycelium, which lacks most of Chaga's active benefits it gets from the trees.

There's a lot of chatter about sustainability and Chaga. Some say it's unsustainable to use wild herbs and mushrooms. This is far from the truth, especially when it comes to Chaga, which only grows on sick or dying trees, not healthy ones. It can take Chaga up to 20 years to mature, at which point both the host tree and the Chaga die together. Wild harvesting Chaga does not mean killing trees. That being said, look for sustainably harvested Chaga to ensure only part of it is taken out so the tree's "death" isn't accelerated and the Chaga can continue to grow for future yields.

Chaga also grows most prominently in the world's largest forest, the Taiga, which has a larger land mass than the United States. The Natural Resources Institute of Finland says Chaga can be found in about 30 percent of trees in northern Finland and Sweden and in about 6 percent of trees in southern Finland and Sweden.[16] One Russian study claims that Chaga can be found on up to 20 percent of trees in the area.[17] Since you need very little Chaga extract every day, there's hardly any evidence it's unsustainable to forage out in the wild as is necessary for a high-quality product.

MUSHROOM EXTRACTION

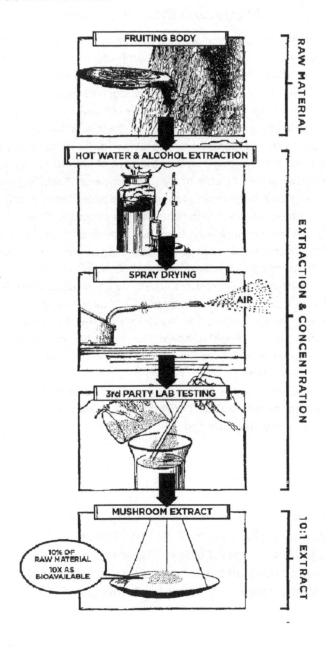

Mushroom Extraction 101

Functional mushrooms contain a compound called *chitin* within their cell walls. It's the same compound found in crustacean shells (think crab, lobster, or shrimp). Chitin acts like a door, blocking your body from being able to reach the beneficial compounds within the mushroom. Thus, breaking through the cell wall via extraction is critical for making the compounds within the functional mushrooms bioavailable to your body. If you consume a mushroom that has not been extracted (typically found in the form of powder or capsule), your body will only be able to use it like insoluble fiber. This is not necessarily bad, but it means you will not be able to access many of the mushroom's incredible benefits. It's just expensive fiber.

There are two main ways to extract a mushroom: via hot water (called a decoction) or alcohol (a tincture). Since some compounds in the mushroom are water soluble and others alcohol soluble, the type of extraction will determine the benefits of the final product. If you want all the beneficial compounds, you will need a double or dual extraction, where the mushroom has been decocted *and* tinctured. This is the gold standard. Dual extraction ensures that all beneficial compounds from the fungi are unlocked and available for your body to utilize.

Warning: there are many mushroom products on the market that are not extracted at all. Avoid them! At minimum, get a product that is hot-water extracted.

When using a wild-harvested Chaga that has been dual extracted, start with 500 to 1,500 milligrams per day. Benefits begin to plateau around 3,000 milligrams per day, so use that as the maximum daily allotment. Always start with small doses and increase slowly based on your body's feedback.

REAL-LIFE WAYS TO BENEFIT FROM CHAGA

- *For immunity:* As an antioxidant-rich immune supplement to be sipped daily during the winter season

- *For longevity:* As a caffeine-free coffee alternative with a splash of plant milk and cinnamon daily for overall well-being

- *For beauty:* Add a scoop of powdered extract to your travel mug to protect your skin (from the inside out) from sun damage on your next tropical vacation.

Defend *(Immunity and Protection)* Case Study

At the young age of 31, a woman wrote to tell us her story of being diagnosed with stage 3 breast cancer. She was "in the fight for [her] life," pursuing all means necessary to heal. She went through conventional treatment, which killed the cancer but left her with a lot of physical and emotional pain. Due to her age and the severity of the cancer, she was told that there was a high probability of recurrence. After the initial treatments, she found herself in a fragile place of trying to heal while also working to strengthen her system enough to prevent any future recurrences.

A few years after treatment, she started using a blend of Adaptogenic functional mushroom extracts, including Chaga. This blend of functional mushroom Adaptogens has been her go-to daily supplement to support her health and wellness for several years. Physically, her renewed energy has enabled her to start a weight-lifting routine. Mentally, she has improved clarity and memory, which has been incredibly helpful to her as a writer and editor who previously suffered from "chemo brain." She credits her success in large part to her Adaptogenic mushroom regimen.

ELEUTHERO

Full legal name: *Eleutherococcus senticosus* (Chinese botanists refer to it as *Acanthopanax senticosus*), in the Araliaceae family

Nicknames: Russian root, taiga root, Wucha, Siberian Ginseng (although it's not a real Ginseng!)

Power hub: Root (the stem and bark have also been used in traditional medicine systems)

Home: Northern mountains of China and Russia

Energetics: Warm, dry

Helpful with:

1. Immunity
2. Endurance
3. Brain health

Comes with:

- Eleutherosides C, D, B (syringin), E (syringaresinol)
- Triterpenoid saponins
- Coumarins
- Polysaccharides
- Flavonoid compounds
- Caffeic acid, isofraxidin, glycosides

Common uses: Provides a surge of energy when you're feeling tired and sluggish

Best friends: Chaga, Schisandra, Rhodiola, and echinacea

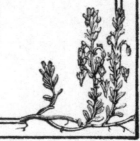

A BRIEF HISTORY: From East to West

Eleuthero was the first plant coined an Adaptogen, although it was used for 2,000 years before it received the "Adaptogen" label. Eleuthero was first written about in Traditional Chinese Medicine's oldest pharmacopeia. Chinese herbalist Li Shih-chen wrote, "I would rather have a handful of Wucha [Eleuthero] than a cartload of gold and jewels." It was known for its spicy and stimulating properties, particularly helpful for joint pain.

Russian researchers can be thanked for bringing Eleuthero to the West. On their quest to find the most powerful substances on the planet, they came across Eleuthero. They studied its effects in over two thousand people in trials spanning several decades and found that it significantly increased people's resistance to stressors, including workload.[18] It also improved stamina and recovery, oxygen intake, and performance in athletes.

Due to the success of these early Russian studies, Eleuthero's use continued. It was given to people in Chernobyl to help their bodies combat the physical stress of radiation. It was also prescribed to Soviet Union cosmonauts and people in the Soyuz space program. Turns out, Eleuthero is so powerful that it can protect against the effects of zero gravity on the body!

HELPFUL WITH IMMUNITY

One of Eleuthero's most traditional uses is as an immune ally to prevent colds and flus. The main compounds interacting with our body's immune system are Eleutherosides, which *activate innate immunity*. This is your body's first line of immune defense. Increased innate immunity means you are less prone to getting sick in the first place. It also gives your body defenses against acute illnesses.

A double-blind, placebo-controlled study found that the group given Eleuthero had a "drastic increase" in immunocompetent cells and improved T lymphocytes, important white blood cells that protect against pathogens. They also improved cytotoxic T cells, a type of lymphocyte that protects against toxicity, as well as natural killer cells, lymphocytes that play a major role in fighting virally infected cells.[19]

Eleuthero, especially when used with other herbs, has clinically proven benefits. Another double-blind, placebo-controlled study looked at the combination of Eleuthero and Andrographis. Andrographis (sometimes called "Indian echinacea") is an herb used in Ayurvedic medicine for its immune benefits. When both herbs were taken within 72 hours of the first symptoms of a cold, the severity and length of the cold were reduced.[20]

HELPFUL WITH ENDURANCE

Eleuthero helps the body perform for long periods of time without burnout or exhaustion. It's been widely studied in Russia and China for its performance-enhancing properties and has also been clinically proven to help combat physical stressors. In a study examining water extracts of five Eleutherosides from Eleuthero, Eleutherosides C, D, and E were found to significantly prolong rats' swimming time. Furthermore, D and E reduced corticosterone levels (which are often indicative of inflammation), while Eleutheroside E showed anti-fatigue action amidst the stress of prolonged swimming.[21]

It's again important to remember that the sum is greater than the parts. When it comes to Eleuthero, like all Adaptogens, it's not just one compound that offers benefits. Eleutherosides are just one group of phytochemicals that positively affect your body. One eight-week study with athletic males found that Eleuthero improves stamina through better use of lipids and spare glycogen.[22] This leads to reduced lactic acid buildup, increased oxygen, and better use of energy (blood glucose and lipid utilization).[23] Eleuthero is among the safest and most effective herbs for serious athletes and weekend warriors alike.

HELPFUL FOR THE BRAIN

Eleuthero has long been touted for its effects on the brain and memory. It can help fight mental fatigue, improve concentration, and elevate mood. This may be due to its Eleutherosides, which have shown regenerative effects on neural synapses in rat brains.[24] Researchers have also found significant improvement in axonal and dendritic regeneration with Eleuthero. Eleutheroside B protected against cell death and supported memory[25] and has demonstrated anti-depressive effects in rat trials.[26]

Several animal studies suggest that at one to two grams per kilogram of body weight per day, Eleuthero helps to increase levels of serotonin, epinephrine, and dopamine, the neurotransmitters that regulate depression, mood, and pleasure in our brain.[27,28]

PREPARATION, SOURCING, AND DOSAGE

There are a lot of mislabeled Eleuthero products on the market. Be sure to buy products that are made from true *Eleutherococcus senticosus*. Many products labeled Eleuthero or Siberian Ginseng are not the real *senticosus* species. A good quick test is to see if the key constituents, Eleutherosides, are called out on the product. Our recommended dosage is one to three grams per day (about 1/2 teaspoon) in a powder form, or 50 to 100 drops up to three times per day in a tincture.

We've seen the best results when starting small. Continually assess how your body is responding after you first take it. After about a week at a low dose, you can slowly increase it as your body needs. Then either increase or decrease your dose accordingly.

REAL-LIFE WAYS TO BENEFIT FROM ELEUTHERO

- *For immunity:* Take during immune-vulnerable times like the change of seasons or at the first sign of an ailment.

- *For endurance:* If you're an athlete, take in the recovery period of training. It can also be used before a big trip where jetlag is likely.

- *For brain:* Use instead of coffee or caffeinated beverages in the morning or midday to lift your energy.

TURKEY TAIL

Full legal name: *Trametes versicolor* from the large *Polyporaceae* family. It has two Latin names: *coriolus* is typically used in Asia, and *trametes* in the rest of the world

Nicknames: River mushroom, cloud mushroom, mother of Krestin

Power hub: Mushroom fruiting body

Home: A true nomad, Turkey Tail lives in woodlands across the world

Energetics: Slightly warm, slightly dry

Helpful with:

1. Immunity
2. Gut Health
3. Longevity

Comes with:

- Polysaccharide K (PSK)
- Polysaccharide P (PSP)
- Ergosterol
- Vitamin D

Common uses: Helps to digest meals, with changes of season, and serves as your cheerleader during cold and flu season

Best friends: Reishi, Chaga, shiitake, maitake, rose hips, and warming spices like cinnamon and ginger

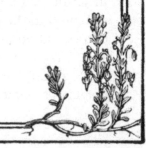

A BRIEF HISTORY: The Best-Selling
Anti-Cancer Drug in Japan

In the wild, this astounding mushroom resembles the flared tail of a turkey, hence its common name. In Asian cultures, it's called "cloud mushroom" since clouds symbolize longevity and spiritual fulfillment. Its use as a medicinal tea is recorded as early as the Ming dynasty in the 15th century. It's been used for three thousand years in China, Asia, and Europe, and among indigenous tribes of Native America. Laplanders of Finland used it as an aphrodisiac. In Mexico, it was used to treat impetigo and ringworm. The Chinese used it for increasing circulation and treating fevers, and Malaysians used it to treat dysentery. Natives of North and South Dakota discovered that enzymes in Turkey Tail were able to bleach garments. Aborigines of Australia sucked on the mushroom to treat mouth sores. And externally, it's been used for skin conditions like eczema.

Turkey Tail is one of the easiest functional mushrooms to spot out in the wild. It's abundant in almost all forested ecosystems on earth and is often found growing on pine trees, which are evergreen and never lose their leaves. Taoists believed the mushrooms would collect *yang* energy from the pine. Yang is the positive, bright, and masculine principle in Chinese philosophy. It's associated with light, power, vitality, and strength. So by consuming Turkey Tail, it is thought the yang energy is passed on to the person who ingests the mushroom.

Turkey Tail is one of the most researched of all functional mushrooms. It is also a prime example of how many pharmaceuticals are derived from nature. In 1965, a chemical engineer working for Kureha Corporation, a chemical industry company in Japan, had a neighbor with late-stage gastric cancer that had advanced to the point where he was rejected for treatment at all clinics and hospitals. He attempted to cure himself using Turkey Tail. After a few months of daily consumption, he went back to work, completely cured. The engineer was blown away by his neighbor's miraculous recovery and convinced his company to study the mushroom. They identified two potent water-soluble anti-cancer polysaccharides. One was named polysaccharide K (PSK)—with the *K* for "Kureha," the company that discovered it.[29] PSK became the first mushroom-derived cancer drug approved by the Japanese government.

HELPFUL WITH IMMUNITY

A potent immunomodulator, Turkey Tail is best known for its immune supportive properties. While PSK is now deemed an anti-cancer drug, the whole-mushroom extract (remember how important synergy is!) is used in *conjunction* with conventional cancer therapies. The mushroom extract reboots the immune system in depleted states, though we like to think of Turkey Tail as boot camp for the immune system, no matter what stage of fitness it's at.

A meta-analysis that looked at 13 gold standard studies of Turkey Tail and cancer patients found that when Turkey Tail is used as an adjunct therapy, there is a significant increase in survival rates. It was especially effective in breast, gastric, and colorectal cancers.[30] Another meta-analysis covering eight thousand patients from eight randomized trials showed that after cancerous tissue was removed, PSK became particularly useful. Here, the combination of PSK and chemotherapy significantly improved survival rates.[31]

Turkey Tail's polysaccharides have also been shown to reduce general symptoms of sickness. Extracts have been found to increase macrophages "7.2-fold over controls."[32]

HELPFUL WITH GUT HEALTH

Today, gut health is a very popular field of research, as it has been shown to be an important indicator of immunity, skin health, and mood. We're discovering the vital importance of the microbiome on nearly every system in the body. A key component of a healthy gut is the balance and diversity of microorganisms that reside within the microbiome. Probiotics have become a household word, but prebiotics are newer to most.

As you may guess from the prefix, *prebiotics* act as food for *probiotics*. Polysaccharides from Turkey Tail, specifically PSP, act as a powerful prebiotic. In an eight-week study, the group given PSP had clear and consistent microbiome changes in comparison to groups given antibiotics and no treatment, proving PSP's prebiotic activity.[33] Another human study showed that Turkey Tail polysaccharides increased bifidobacterium and lactobacillus species, both "good bacteria" that are beneficial for a healthy gut. The extract also reduced dangerous bacterial species.[34,35,36,37]

HELPFUL WITH LONGEVITY

Turkey Tail is a superhero when it comes to supporting two of the body's most foundational systems key to helping prevent body deterioration: the immune and gastrointestinal (GI) systems. Beyond its polysaccharides, this mushroom also contains other powerful compounds that are allies to longevity, including ergosterol. Ergosterol is the precursor to both vitamins D2 and D3. Similar to our human skin, Turkey Tail turns ergosterol into vitamin D when exposed to UV light. Vitamin D is critical to a healthy immune system, gut, and healthy aging. Ample levels of vitamin D help extend our lifespan. A study from the Buck Institute for Research on Aging showed that an inadequate level of serum vitamin D may be foundational to a wide variety of human age-related diseases. Conversely, sufficient levels of vitamin D are a key component to anti-aging.[38]

Turkey Tail is also packed with antioxidants. As you know by now, antioxidants are vital to keeping your body free from chronic inflammation and the many side effects of aging. Antioxidants in Turkey Tail help reduce the damage from oxidative stress. Antioxidants unique to Turkey Tail are the flavonoids quercetin and baicalein, plus a range of phenols. Current research shows there may be as many as 35 unique phenolic compounds in Turkey Tail fruiting bodies.[39] These phenols show protective effects against many of the most common ailments in today's world, including cancer, heart disease, GI issues, and neurodegenerative diseases like Alzheimer's.[40]

PREPARATION, SOURCING, AND DOSAGE

As with all functional mushrooms, it's best to use the fruiting body grown from the wood it natively grows on. When it comes to Turkey Tail, this can mean wild harvested or log-grown mushrooms. In addition, remember that extraction is always critical to ensure the compounds in the mushrooms are bioavailable to your body. Since PSP and PSK are both polysaccharides, and sugars are hydrophobic, or water-soluble (think how easily sugar mixes with water), the best way to extract these beneficial compounds is via decoction.

If you are making your own decoction from wild Turkey Tail mushrooms, we suggest decocting in a crockpot for several hours (six to eight hours is ideal). Use one part Turkey Tail fruiting body to 10 parts water. Alternatively, Turkey Tail can also be found in an ethanol or alcohol extract, which can also be beneficial. As with all functional mushrooms, the gold standard is to use a dual extraction for maximum benefits.

A typical dose of Turkey Tail ranges from 500 to 1,500 milligrams per day. In cancer patients, the dosage may be as high as six grams per day during the treatment period. If taking PSP and PSP as isolated extracts, take dosages of one to two grams each as a preventative measure. With a serious healing protocol, use up to six grams per day, remembering to take breaks (for example two weeks on, two weeks off).

REAL-LIFE WAYS TO BENEFIT FROM TURKEY TAIL

- *For immunity:* Use in a blend of other functional mushroom extracts to support the immune system in vulnerable times.

- *For gut health:* Add to coffee, black tea, or chai for a gut-supportive, prebiotic rich beverage.

- *For longevity:* Add the powdered extract into smoothies for overall well-being.

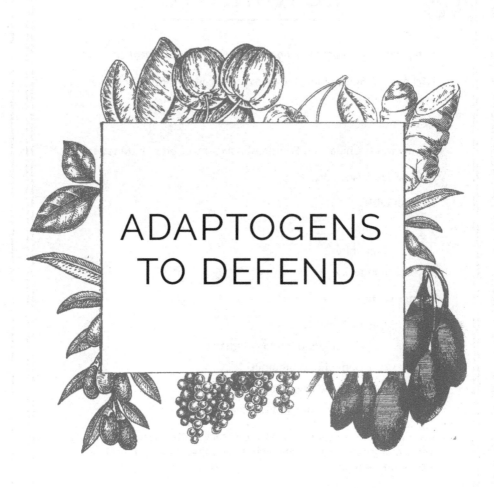

ADAPTOGENS TO DEFEND

FOR BEAUTY AND SKIN

TURMERIC

Full legal name: *Curcuma longa* from the ginger (*Zingiberaceae*) family

Nicknames: Spice of life, Indian saffron, yellow ginger, and over 50 Sanskrit names

Power hub: Root

Home: India, China, and Southeast Asia—most often Indonesia

Energetics: Warm, dry

Helpful with:

1. Beauty
2. Immunity
3. Longevity

Comes with:

- Curcumininoids
    - Curcumin (diferuloylmethane)
    - Demethoxycurcumin
    - Bisdemethoxycurcumin
- Oils: Zingiberene and turmerone

Common uses: Getting you back on track at the early signs of any inflammatory symptoms (headaches, digestive issues, sniffles) morning, noon, or night

Best friends: Turkey Tail, black pepper, ginger, coconut, cinnamon, and honey

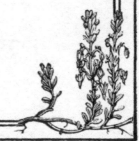

A BRIEF HISTORY: The Golden Root
from Ayurveda to America

This bright orange root has been used as a spice, dye, food, and medicine across India and Asia for over 4,000 years. Ancient pots discovered near Delhi had 2,500-year-old residues of Turmeric, ginger, and garlic on them. Turmeric was first recorded as medicine in the year 659 in the Vedic *Tang Materia Medica*. In India, the world's largest producer of Turmeric, it's a staple in daily life. It is used as a key ingredient in curries and externally for skin ailments, including acne, burns, psoriasis, and shingles. In Ayurveda, Turmeric is a remedy for digestive issues and nausea, which isn't surprising given that it's a cousin to ginger. The root is also seen as auspicious and sacred. In India, Turmeric has been worn around the neck to protect from evil spirits and is a part of wedding ceremonies, where a string is dyed with Turmeric and placed around the bride's neck by her groom as a symbol of marriage. The beautiful golden hue is also used as a dye to create the vibrant color of Buddhist robes.

It may be safe to say that Turmeric is the second best-known and used Adaptogen in the modern West, right after Cacao. After the British colonized India, they brought Turmeric to the West. Yet it wasn't until the last few decades that it gained popularity for its medicinal benefits. With the rising interest in inflammation, modern research around Turmeric skyrocketed. Its key constituent, curcumin, is a powerful antioxidant. Discovered in 1842 by two German scientists, curcumin has been included in over four thousand studies for its health benefits.[1] It's now recommended for beauty, immunity, and longevity around the world and might even rival the anti-inflammatory properties found in drugs such as Ibuprofen.

HELPFUL WITH BEAUTY

One of the many names for Turmeric in Sanskrit is matrimanika, which translates to "as beautiful as the moonlight." In nearly all anti-aging products, antioxidants are front and center. This is because antioxidants are the main defense to combat dangerous free radicals. Unfortunately, free radicals are unavoidable, since they occur on a daily basis through exposure to such things as the sun and toxins, and through the aging process. Without antioxidants, these free radicals cause cellular damage, which can lead to tissue death, organ dysfunction, and diseases, including cancer. Enter the super antioxidant root, Turmeric. It supports beauty and healthy skin from the inside out and outside in. Hundreds of studies confirm curcumin's anti-inflammatory, antimicrobial, and antibacterial dermatological benefits.[2,3]

HELPFUL WITH IMMUNITY

Curcumin is immunomodulatory, meaning it can stimulate or suppress immune activity based on individual needs. It modulates the activity of T cells, B cells, macrophages, neutrophils, natural killer (NK) cells, and dendritic cells.[4] It can also down-regulate the expression of various proinflammatory cytokines. This suggests it may be beneficial in inflammatory disorders, including arthritis, allergies, heart disease, Alzheimer's disease, and even cancer.

Beyond its immunomodulation and anti-inflammatory capabilities, it has also shown antiviral activity.[5] It's a proven antimutagenic, protecting DNA from oxidative stress. In a randomized controlled trial conducted in West Bengal, India, participants exposed to arsenic contamination from groundwater were given daily doses of Turmeric. After three months, DNA damage was reduced, and the oxidative stress of body fats slowed down. This confirmed curcumin's protective role against DNA damage caused by arsenic.[6]

HELPFUL WITH LONGEVITY

Chronic inflammation is the common denominator in many major ailments today. Acute inflammation is a necessary biological function short term. However, issues begin to arise when inflammation becomes chronic. Prolonged inflammation can lead to fatigue, immune suppression, skin issues, heart disease, and more. Modern lifestyle, diet, and the state of our environment are just a few factors that contribute to the inflammatory state most of us are living in. Addressing inflammation is critical to allowing your body to heal from disease.

Turmeric is one of nature's strongest anti-inflammatories, primarily due to curcuminoids, one of three polyphenols in the root. The most studied and active curcuminoid is curcumin, which down-regulates inflammation and aggressive cytokines, inhibiting several molecules that play a role in inflammation. This makes it a great ally for addressing cardiovascular, metabolic, and neurological diseases.[7,8]

PREPARATION, SOURCING, AND DOSAGE

There's a lot of Turmeric out on the market, so there are a few key things to look for to ensure you are getting a good quality supplement. Although long-term benefits can be achieved with regular low usage of powdered Turmeric, best results are typically seen from Turmeric that has been standardized to 95 percent curcumin. Some herbalists we know have seen effective results with prolonged, consistent use of the simple powder, but if possible, look for an extract. This will automatically exclude Turmeric you'd find in the spice aisle, which is typically powdered root rather than an extract.

There is a wide variety of Turmeric products on the market that range drastically in terms of quality, and Turmeric more than most other Adaptogens can contain heavy amounts of pesticides. As such, purity is vitally important here. The best way to assess purity is through third-party laboratory testing. If this isn't clear on a label, reach out to the company. If they do third-party testing of their ingredients, they will usually be willing to share their findings. Look for products that have been tested and cleared for things like heavy metals, herbicides, and pesticides.

Finally, be sure to always add black pepper to any Turmeric you're ingesting. *Pipera nigra* (black pepper) enhances the absorption of curcumin in your body by up to 2,000 percent.[9] If using an extracted root powder, an effective daily dose is one gram or about quarter of a teaspoon. Larger dosages are still safe,[10] but not necessary if you combine Turmeric with black pepper. You can also try mixing Turmeric with black pepper in high-quality organic honey or coconut oil. Add half a teaspoon of the infused oil or honey into tea, dressings, or soups.

Many grocery stores now sell the full fresh Turmeric root as well, which is great for cooking or juicing. If using fresh Turmeric, remember that the fresh root is much less potent than an extract. A daily recommended dose of the fresh root is between 1.5 and 3 grams per day. Whatever form you decide to use, remember to use it regularly to receive noticeable health benefits.

REAL-LIFE WAYS TO BENEFIT FROM TURMERIC

- *For beauty:* Combine with black pepper and sprinkle on anything and everything savory you cook to keep your skin glowing from the inside out. (You can also use it topically with a base oil and apply consistently for a range of dermatological benefits.)

- *For immunity:* Make golden honey or golden oil by mixing Turmeric and black pepper into high-quality honey or coconut oil. Add to tea, soups, smoothies, or take a spoonful when your immune system needs a pick-me-up.

- *For longevity:* Mix Turmeric with black pepper and warming, carminative spices like ginger, a touch of sweetness like honey, and your favorite plant-based milk for DIY golden milk as a longevity tonic.

Defend *(Beauty and Skin)* Case Study

A young man in his twenties with an autoimmune condition presented with severe digestive issues from chronic inflammation in his GI. He was scheduled to begin a strong prescription medication, which he strongly wanted to avoid due to the many side effects of the drug. This is when he came to Danielle with a six-month timeline. They immediately started to build up his diet, fueling his system with the nutrients his body needed to reduce inflammation and start healing. Food sensitivities that were triggering inflammation were fully removed. He started an herbal formula focused on gut health, immune support, and reducing inflammation, the key ingredient being Turmeric (plus black pepper, of course). While there were many contributing factors to the reduction of inflammation and profound gut healing (primarily due to his compliance, commitment, and the support of the herbal allies and dietary changes), within the six-month timeline, his inflammation was reduced to the point that he did not need to go onto the suggested immunosuppressant medication. Thanks, Turmeric!

GOJI

Full legal name: *Lycium barbarum/chinense* from the nightshade (*Solanaceae*) family

Nicknames: Miracle berry, wolfberry, matrimony vine, and red diamond

Power hub: The fruit, specifically the berries

Home: Originally Tibet, but now primarily China and Mongolia

Energetics: Neutral temperature, slightly moist

Helpful with:

1. Beauty
2. Immunity
3. Libido

Comes with:

- Antioxidants: carotenoids, flavonoids, zeaxanthin, and lutein
- Sesquiterpenes
- Polysaccharides
- 18 amino acids (a whole protein)
- Vitamins B1, B2, B6, A, and C
- 22 minerals, including zinc, iron, copper, calcium, potassium, selenium, sodium, phosphorus, magnesium, germanium, and manganese

Common uses: After meals and before you're gearing up to get it on

Best friends: Cacao, Maca, Gynostemma, mulberry, licorice, cashews, mint

A BRIEF HISTORY: From the Oldest
Man on Earth to a Modern Superfruit

Small but mighty, Goji has been a symbol of both youth and longevity for thousands of years. Known as "the berry that keeps you looking long," Goji has legends almost as old as time. It's believed to hold wisdom about life; its Latin name *lycium* means "school of learning." At the same time, throughout its five-thousand-year cultivation history, Goji has been said to be the secret to longevity.

Li Ching-Yuen, a Chinese herbalist, claimed to have lived for 256 years (from 1677 to 1933)! He supposedly lectured at Peking University when he was over 200. Although his age claims sound highly unrealistic, he attributed his great eyesight, posture, and energy at a very old age (even if it was "only" 100 years old) to spring water, daily exercises, and a daily tea of Goji, Ginseng, and Reishi. Another legend tells of a Chinese doctor who visited a village where everyone was over 100 years old. Searching for how this could be possible, he walked around the village and found a well overgrown with Goji vines, where the ripe berries would fall into the well, steep in the water, and create a nutrient-rich Goji tea that the villagers drank from. A true elixir of youth!

Old stories have only propelled Goji's entrance into the modern-day mainstream. It's now renowned as a superfood sold at health food stores and found on menus at high-end restaurants. Modern research confirms that Goji helps with anti-aging, immunity, eyesight, kidney health, and liver health.[11]

HELPFUL WITH BEAUTY

Most beauty products tout high amounts of Vitamins C, Vitamin B, or antioxidants. Goji has it all, and more. First, it's a complete protein with 16 amino acids. It contains six vitamins, 22 minerals, omega fatty acids, and beta-carotene. Goji has 500 times more vitamin C ounce for ounce than oranges. Vitamin C protects the skin from sun damage and wrinkles, boosts collagen production, and diminishes scars.

Another reason Goji is a beauty berry is because of its rich antioxidant profile. In a randomized, double-blind, placebo-controlled study, a 30-day clinical trial found that antioxidant markers significantly increased in those taking Goji compared to the placebo group, showing antioxidants are effective in preventing oxidative stress.[12]

HELPFUL WITH IMMUNITY

One of your body's keys to longevity is a steady production of human growth hormone (HGH), which is vital to the regeneration of our brain and vital organs throughout our entire life. Insufficient amounts of HGH are linked to lowered libido, energy loss, baldness, and memory loss, and sufficient HGH is associated with hair growth, skin tightening, weight loss, increased energy, strong bones, strong libido, better sleep, and improved mood.[13] You may have heard about bodybuilders getting their hands on synthetic HGH to increase muscle mass. Goji's amino acids, vitamins, and minerals naturally boost HGH. It also contains sesquiterpenes that stimulate the pineal and pituitary glands to increase the production of L-glutamine and L-arginine, all of which increases the production of HGH.

HGH is a hormonal lead domino that influences the function of many other hormones. It is critical in aging because, as your body grows older, the amount of HGH produced decreases. A 70-year-old body only makes 10 percent of the HGH of a 20-year-old body. This may be a key reason for Goji's connection to youth and longevity.

Goji has long been touted for its immune benefits, likely due to the Lycium berry polysaccharides (LBPs) it contains. In a randomized, double-blind, placebo-controlled study, participants who ingested 120 milliliters of Goji juice per day showed a significant increase in several key immune markers (like lymphocytes and immunoglobulin G) versus the placebo group that showed no changes in any immune measures. The Goji group also had less fatigue, better sleep, and improved short-term memory, all without negative side effects or adverse reactions.[14]

HELPFUL WITH LIBIDO

Beyond being immunomodulatory, the LBPs in Goji directly interact with the male reproductive system. LBPs increase the quantity, quality, and motility of sperm count. They also protect the testes against accumulating a toxic load, which can lead to sexual problems.

Furthermore, Goji's antioxidants show a positive effect on erectile dysfunction. In a 2017 study out of Seoul, Korea, 24 elderly rats were divided into three groups. One group took a placebo, the second group was given 150 milligrams per kilogram of body weight per day of Goji extract, and the third group received 300 milligrams per kilogram per day. After six weeks, the test subjects' weight, testosterone, antioxidant, nitric oxide (NO)/cyclic guanosine monophosphate–related parameters (GMP), and blood pressure were examined. Multiple markers were needed because scientific testing for erection is much less linear than in the wild! Both groups treated with Goji had increased serum testosterone levels and blood flow. This showed that Goji extract has positive effects on erectile dysfunction.[15]

We can also attribute some of Goji's libido supportive action to LBPs.

PREPARATION, SOURCING, AND DOSAGE

Goji is often treated with chemicals like sulfur dioxide, a toxic gas that irritates skin, lungs, and the mucous membranes of your body. Look for minimally processed Goji that has not been exposed to high heat to ensure the maximum amount of nutrients are left intact. As with many other Adaptogens, it's also important that they have not been radiated in customs when entering the West. If you have high-quality, organic, and minimally processed Goji, their utility is vast. You can boil them in soups or tea for a more traditional experience or add them into trail mix or raw chocolate. Some brands claim to offer "fresh Goji," but it's more likely that additional moisture was added to dried Goji before packing. If you get a good source, dried Goji are just fine. Get creative with how to use them and have fun!

REAL-LIFE WAYS TO BENEFIT FROM GOJI

- *For beauty:* Steep as a tea and drink daily to support skin health and a youthful glow.

- *For immunity:* Add to soups as a touch of sweetness (traditionally used in rice soups, but today added to many broths) to keep your immune system strong during flu season or as the weather turns.

- *For libido:* Take a handful of dried berries as a snack before getting it on.

SCHISANDRA

Full legal name: *Schisandra chinensis* from the *Schisandraceae* family

Nickname: Five-flavor berry, Chinese magnolia vine

Power hub: Traditionally just the seeds, now the full berry

Home: Northern China, Russia, and Korea, and occasionally Hawaii and the Northeast US

Energetics: "Amphoteric"; can be cool and moist or warm and dry

Helpful with:

1. Beauty
2. Endurance
3. Stress

Comes with:

- Lignans
  - ¤ Schisandrin B (also contains alpha-, gamma-, delta-, and deoxyschisandrin)
  - ¤ Gomisin A (also gomisin N)
  - ¤ Schizandrol A
- Triterpenoids
- Vitamin C
- Vitamin E
- Antioxidants

Common uses: Mornings, traveling, and all kinds of exercise (particularly cross-country skiing)

Best friends: All other super berries plus Rhodiola, Eleuthero, and Cordyceps

A BRIEF HISTORY: How the Five-Flavor Berry Became a Nationally Recognized Drug

In traditional systems of medicine, taste plays a key role in the medicinal value of a plant or fungi. Spiciness offers warmth to your body. Saltiness brings mineral and nutrient-rich qualities. Sourness stimulates digestion. Bitterness cools, stimulates, and aids in detoxification. Sweetness boosts energy levels. Schisandra is the only Adaptogen (and natural medicine, for that matter!) that encompasses all five flavors, which provides a unique balancing effect on multiple systems of the body. Its name in TCM, wu wei zi, translates to "five-flavor berry."

Schisandra was first documented two thousand years ago in the Chinese Materia Medica Shen Nong's *Herbal Classic*. It has also been used as a key medicinal in Ayurveda and as a tonic in Korea and Japan. Traditionally, the seed was used to relieve fatigue, improve stamina, and increase energy levels. The seed was also used as an astringent—an herbal action that helps to tonify overly moist tissue states. Today, most people use the whole berry or an extract of it.

Some of the earliest stories of humans using Schisandra stem from wild Nanai hunters. They would bring handfuls of dried berries with them on long treks across Siberia. Chewing on the seeds kept their energy high, stress low, improved night vision, and reduced hunger. In the early 1960s, the Russian government became aware of Chinese clinical research and proven benefits of the berry.[16] They made the seed extract an official medicine in the national pharmacopoeia of the U.S.S.R., and it is still a registered medicine in Russia today, primarily used for vision problems. Besides Eleuthero and Rhodiola, Schisandra is one of the first "official" Adaptogens in the world.

HELPFUL WITH BEAUTY

Clinical trials show that Schisandra contains antioxidants beneficial for skin health, protective against UV radiation, and perhaps most notably, supportive of liver detoxification.

Supporting lasting beauty comes from the inside out, which often means beginning with the liver. The liver is our largest internal organ. It's responsible for hundreds of mechanisms in your body but can simply be thought of as your body's filter. Without filtration of toxins, blockage occurs. Exposure to toxins is inevitable. It happens daily through food, water, and air. Thus, ensuring that these toxins have a way to get out of your body is essential. Without the outlet of the liver, these toxins escape to other porous areas of your body, like the skin, where it can result in acne, eczema, and psoriasis.

Schisandra demonstrates hepatoprotective (liver-supportive) properties. It helps regenerate hepatocytes (liver cells) and increases hepatic (liver) glutathione. It protects the liver from being damaged by things like drugs and promotes the healing of existing damage. As an Adaptogen, it also protects against stress-induced liver damage. This helps create lasting holistic beauty.[17]

HELPFUL WITH ENDURANCE

Schisandra berries have an age-old reputation of providing anti-fatigue benefits. These traditional benefits are now further supported by modern research.[18] A true performance berry, it uses the classic push/pull action of Adaptogens. Schisandra calms anxiety, keeping your body from burning out, while simultaneously increasing energy. This gentle stimulation offers a lift in energy and a decrease in fatigue without a crash later.

Schisandra has been called a "Qi invigorator."[19,20] It has an affinity for the lungs, helping to deepen and even the breathing. Control of breathing positively affects your heart rate and ability to endure a workout. These two properties also make Schisandra a sexual enhancer, another type of endurance. Schisandra supports the body during and after an endurance performance with protective effects on exercise-induced stress in recovery.

Intense physical exercise increases the content of nitric oxide (NO) and cortisol. Nitric oxide is a free radical. Cortisol is the central stress hormone. These are both things you do not want in your bloodstream for extended periods of time. In one double-blind, placebo-controlled study, participants who took an Adaptogen extract of Schisandra and bryonia had no increase in nitric oxide or cortisol, while the placebo group exhibited increased NO. This shows the stress-positive effect of Schisandra in endurance and Schisandra's aptitude for supporting performance and recovery.[21]

HELPFUL WITH STRESS

Schisandra has a unique effect on the nervous system. Its premier ability to combat stress is part of what makes it beneficial for performance and beauty. Like all Adaptogens, it interacts with the nervous, immune, and endocrine systems. But it has a dual effect on the central nervous system. It both stimulates reflexes and mental activity while also calming and relieving anxiety. It's helpful for conditions like stress-induced asthma because of its effects on the nervous system and lungs. A steady and even breath rate is not just important for performance. Proper breathing is also key to keeping your body out of long-term stress. Prolonged shallow and rapid breathing can lead to panic and heart palpitations. Schisandra helps to keep the lungs calm and steady and allows an even and sufficient flow of oxygen.

Schisandra fruit and seed extract have been shown to produce mood-enhancing effects when taken for 16 to 40 days and to inhibit nervous system exhaustion, gland atrophy, and depression in animal models.[22]

PREPARATION, SOURCING, AND DOSAGE

While Schisandra is mostly sold in the West as a whole dried berry, most of the traditional research is done on the seed extract. One of the key constituents in Schisandra, schisandrins, are mostly found in the seed. That said, an extract of the whole fruit or seed will result in beneficial effects. If using crude berries, start with three to six grams decocted for at least 10 to 20 minutes. The dried berry-to-water ratio should be 1:20 (weight/volume) and consumed in doses of five ounces up to twice per day.

The Russian pharmacopoeia and Traditional Chinese Medicine share this same recommendation as a general Schisandra preparation. If using a tincture, we recommend starting with about 30 drops or 1 milliliter twice per day. A high-quality and potent tincture should be made with dried fruits at 1:6 (weight/volume) using 95 percent ethanol. As a standardized extract in powder, look for 9 percent Schisandrins for the highest potency. Start with 400 to 500 milligrams with a maximum dosage of two grams per day. To narrow it down a bit, we've found that a daily dose of 500 to 1,500 milligrams taken twice per day is a key range for most people. Since Schisandra may boost energy, take it in the morning or midafternoon as a pick-me-up. If sensitive, avoid taking it too late in the day so it doesn't interfere with sleep.

REAL-LIFE WAYS TO BENEFIT FROM SCHISANDRA

- *For beauty:* Make into a decoction and sip daily as part of your beauty routine.
- *For endurance:* Drink as a tea before a long endurance activity (workouts, traveling, or staying up late) or midday as an ally for siesta sex.
- *For stress:* Combine the powder with raw chocolate and nibble when you are having a stressful day.

ACEROLA

Full legal name: *Malpighia emarginata* (previously *Malpighia punicifolia*) from the Barbados cherry family

Nicknames: Garden cherry, Indian cherry, Surinam cherry, or Puerto Rico cherry

Power hub: Fruit

Home: Originally from the Yucatan of Southeast Mexico but can now be found in most tropical regions around the world

Energetics: Neutral to warm, neutral

Helpful with:

1. Beauty
2. Immunity
3. Longevity

Comes with:

- Vitamin C
- Bioflavonoids
- Carotenoids (like lutein, beta-carotene, and beta-cryptoxanthin)
- Anthocyanins
- Minerals (magnesium, potassium, copper, zinc, and iron)
- Vitamin A
- B vitamins (namely B5)

Common uses: Mornings, prepping for photo shoots, and helping with recovery from surgeries

Best friends: Cacao, pomegranate, blueberries, tremella, and mint

A BRIEF HISTORY: The Untapped Functional Superfood

Acerola is a small fruit that grows in almost all tropical and subtropical regions of the world. Nutritionally, it's similar to many other berries and stone fruits. It has a bright color and a bold, sweet, and sharp taste. The berries, skin, and tiny seeds are all edible. Each part of the berry has been consumed as both food and medicine for centuries. It's a delicious fruit eaten raw but traditionally was made into jams and syrups. In modern times, it's used to flavor cocktails and ice cream in South America (Brazil is one of the largest producers of Acerola).

Medicinally, because it contains 50 to 100 times more vitamin C than oranges or lemons, Acerola has been used to prevent vitamin C deficiency and scurvy. Just three small Acerola fruits meet the daily vitamin C requirements of an adult! Vitamin C is also an antioxidant, helping protect your body from free radicals and aiding in building collagen. It helps decrease oxidative damage to important organs like the liver, heart, and brain. As one of the richest natural sources of vitamin C, it's been used to support immune health, vision, skin, digestion, and recovery for millennia.

Acerola is also rich in antioxidants including carotenoids and anthocyanins, which have been revered in kale, carrots, and blueberries. Yet in Acerola, there are much higher amounts of each of these compounds. It also contains an ample amount of vitamin A, another key antioxidant. Each phytochemical present in the cherries works together synergistically. Since it is a food, your body can absorb and utilize its vitamins, antioxidants, and minerals better than synthetic forms of these compounds.

HELPFUL WITH BEAUTY

Acerola's antioxidants help protect the skin from toxins while its vitamin content assists with collagen formation.[23] It even contains the mineral copper, which promotes skin firmness and elastin development. Phytonutrients in Acerola like carotenoids, anthocyanins, and flavonoids are true allies for the skin. Carotenoids support a youthful glow, helping the skin to look young and vibrant. As a bonus, they also support eye health and age-related vision disorders. Research shows Acerola enhances skin texture, regenerates flawed tissue, and slows down aging. It further protects against wrinkles, fine lines, stretch marks, and helps heal scar tissue.[24]

Anthocyanins are what give the cherries their rich hues of red, purple, and blue. (These are the same compounds found in blueberries, red cabbage, beets, and even red beans.) There are literally hundreds of studies on the connection between anthocyanins and healthy skin, examining their antioxidant, anti-inflammatory, and anti-cancer effects. When it comes to the skin, think of anthocyanins as internal sunscreen. They protect skin from the negative effects of prolonged sun exposure like wrinkles, premature aging, and, in the worst case, cancer.

The flavonoids in Acerola help to protect our skin from UV damage by helping us absorb UV radiation, thus reducing sunburn, aging, and various skin damage caused by excess sun exposure. Other antioxidants in Acerola help cleanse, purify, and eliminate toxins from your body.

HELPFUL WITH IMMUNITY

Acerola's immune support ranges from protecting against the common cold to seasonal allergies, as it has 1.5 to 4.5 grams of vitamin C per 100 grams.[25] To put this into context, that is 30 to 90 times more than strawberries and 38 to 115 times more than grapefruits! Vitamin C encourages the body's production of white blood cells, which are a key part of our body's defense system to fight against infections and viruses. This makes Acerola a superfruit during cold and flu seasons to prevent illness and relieve symptoms. Because of its tannins, Acerola has a particular affinity for respiratory diseases. When these tannins contact the gastrointestinal mucosa, they form a layer that protects the skin from sore throats, reflux, and gastritis. Its phenolic compounds are also antibacterial, giving it an additional angle to target infections.

Antioxidants in Acerola like flavonoids and carotenoids fight free radical damage in our body. Unchecked free radicals can lead to the mutation of healthy cells, including the formation of cancer cells. Acerola has been shown to be an effective supplement for lung cancer patients, slowing down the growth of the cancer mass.[26]

Furthermore, it helps reduce both the frequency and intensity of allergies. This is done by modifying the immune response to the allergen. The stimulation of WBCs also helps here. This response shows Acerola's protective and strengthening effect on the immune response.

HELPFUL WITH RECOVERY

Acerola's pectins, aka heteropolysaccharides (galacturonic acid, arabinose, galactose, xylose, and rhamnose), have been shown effective in supporting recovery. These are also directly anti-fatigue. In the athletic realm, recovery is known to be the most important part of a training regimen. Some coaches go as far as to say that any training is effectively useless without a recovery period. Similar to the profound and often underrated benefits of sleep, recovery enables your muscles to repair themselves and your body to redistribute energy to repair and revitalize other systems in the body, following physical, mental, or emotional exertion.

In a study evaluating Acerola's anti-fatigue effects, trained mice who took Acerola extract for 28 days lengthened their swim time, modified how their energy was used in performance, and had positively affected respiration in exercise and antioxidant status.[27]

Another area where Acerola shines in recovery is due to vitamin C's effect on the adrenals, the glands that produce hormones, help regulate metabolism, blood pressure, the immune system, and stress response. When the body is low in vitamin C, the adrenals burn through more cortisol, which can affect blood pressure and metabolism. Since vitamin C is not naturally synthesized by your body, we need to get it from the foods we eat. To top it off, vitamin C decreases oxidative damage to important organs like the liver, heart, and brain.

Yet beyond vitamin C, Acerola contains a range of B vitamins, including riboflavin, folic acid, and niacin. B vitamins are like cellular energy. They are particularly important for plant-based eaters who may not get enough of this vitamin naturally through their diet. In addition, Acerola's multiple antioxidants are key to restoring compounds that were lost or burned during physical or mental exertion.

PREPARATION, SOURCING, AND DOSAGE

Since Acerola is a fruit, it can be eaten whole, raw, or cooked, just like other varieties of cherries. Even its tiny seeds and peel are edible and offer many health benefits. The fresh fruits can also be frozen and consumed throughout the year. If you don't have access to fresh Acerola cherries, don't worry. It's commonly sold as juice, powder, capsules, or tinctures. You can even find it in topical skin-care products. Most commonly, Acerola is freeze-dried, ground into a powder, and then packaged as a bulk powder or in capsules. Sometimes Vitamin C powder itself is made from Acerola.

We always recommended choosing a powder over a capsule as you can taste for potency, plus the benefits are better delivered to your system when you can taste the flavor. With capsules, it's easier to hide less potent or potentially even rancid ingredients. If you have access to the fresh or frozen fruit, three berries per day is a sufficient dose. If using it as a powder, start with one teaspoon or 3.5 grams per day. In specific situations, such as recovery from surgery or sudden illness, one could increase the dose up to 10 grams per day.

REAL-LIFE WAYS TO BENEFIT FROM ACEROLA

- *For beauty:* Add powder into a tea or eat a handful of fresh cherries daily for skin and anti-aging benefits.

- *For immunity:* Sprinkle powder into oatmeal, plant-based yogurt, or a smoothie for daily immune support or take at the first sign of sniffles to help ward off the ailment before it takes hold.

- *For recovery:* Cook cherries into a porridge (with a sprinkle of cinnamon) for a warming, nutrient-rich breakfast when recovering from an illness.

Morning Smoothie Recipe for Beauty and Protection

Try this delicious plant-based smoothie in the mornings as a way to start enjoying the immune-supporting and beauty-enhancing properties of multiple Adaptogens.

> 12 ounces of cold Chaga decoction (or make 8 ounces of hot Chaga tea and add ice cubes)
>
> 1 cup of frozen berries (like wild blueberries)
>
> 1 serving of vanilla plant protein
>
> 1 teaspoon of Acerola powder
>
> 1 teaspoon of Turmeric powder
>
> Few cracks of whole black pepper or a sprinkle of ground pepper
>
> Sprinkle of sea salt

Mix all ingredients well in a high-speed blender until smooth and creamy. Enjoy!

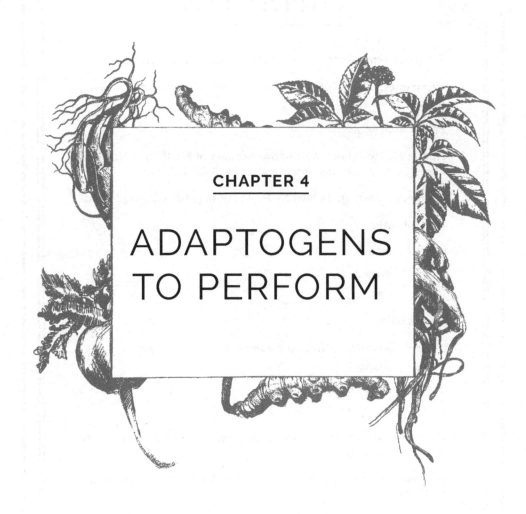

CHAPTER 4

ADAPTOGENS TO PERFORM

FOR ENERGY AND PERFORMANCE

GINSENG

Full legal name: *Panax Ginseng* from the *Araliaceae* family

Nicknames: All-healing root, Asian/Korean/Chinese/Red Ginseng, royal root

Power hub: Root

Home: Nearly extinct in its native habitats of Northern China and Korea, so now cultivated elsewhere across Asia

Energetics: Warm (red Ginseng)/slightly warm (white Ginseng), moist

Helpful with:

1. Energy
2. Libido
3. Brain

Comes with:

*   Ginsenosides (triterpene saponins)
*   Geranium
*   Polysaccharides
*   Antioxidants

Common uses: Being the first to jump out of bed (or staying there all day with a partner)

Best friends: Rhodiola, Cordyceps, Schisandra, Reishi, Ashwagandha, and Tulsi

There are over 400 species of Cordyceps, all with unique characteristics, but most of the history is likely to be with *Ophiocordyceps sinensis*. We now use and recommend its close cousin *Cordyceps militaris* because it's scalable, sustainable, plant-based/vegan, ethical, and equally, if not more medicinal, than the unsustainable *Ophiocordyceps sinensis*.

A BRIEF HISTORY: The Oldest
Known Medicinal Plant

Discovered over five thousand years ago in Northern China, Ginseng may be the oldest known medicinal plant. "Panax" in Greek translates to "all-heal," which is exactly the status Ginseng is elevated to. Chinese emperors valued Ginseng more than gold. At one point, it was forbidden to use unless you were royalty. If a commoner was found with a Ginseng root, it wasn't uncommon to be faced with the penalty of death. There's even a story of three thousand soldiers who were sent on a mission to find wild Ginseng by the first Qin emperor Qin Shi Huang in 221 B.C., and anyone that came back empty-handed was beheaded.

Of all the 11,000-plus herbs in the TCM Materia Medica, Ginseng is known as the king of all Chinese herbs. In the legendary TCM Shen Nong's Materia Medica, it is described as "a tonic to the five viscera (the organs inside your body), quieting the animal spirits, stabilizing the soul, preventing fear, expelling the vicious energies, brightening the eye . . . and prolonging life." At around the same time, it was written about in the Ayurvedic Vedas, a five-thousand-year-old ancient book of scripture from India, as "the root which is dug from the earth and strengthens the nerves. The strength of the horse, the mule, the goat, the ram, moreover the strength of the bull it bestows on him. This herb will make thee so full of lusty strength that thou shalt, when excited, exhale heat as a thing of fire."[1]

Ginseng has a panacea of actions that supports each body uniquely. Famous for its neuroprotective, aphrodisiac, stress-relieving, immunomodulating, and vitality supportive properties, it's a tune-up for the whole body—elevating energy, general health, and longevity.

With the highly revered and almost mystical status of wild Ginseng, it became close to extinct in its native regions. Luckily, it's still cultivated across Asia. It's not just historical lore and praise that give Ginseng its reverence. There are currently over 30,000 studies on this powerful root, proving its support to energy, cognition, stress, and libido.

HELPFUL WITH ENERGY

Ginseng is the most uplifting of all Adaptogens. It is a choice option for people who are exhausted, debilitated, or need a strong kick to get back in gear. It's particularly helpful for people over 40 years old and should be used sparingly by younger individuals who don't yet need its powerfully stimulating action.

In 2016, a meta-analysis of multiple randomized controlled trials on Ginseng and fatigue found statistically significant efficacy of Ginseng supplements in reducing fatigue.[2] In both animal and human trials, Ginseng's multitude of compounds helped to regulate carbohydrate metabolism, protect the brain, and regulate neurotransmitters.[3] One area where Ginseng's energy enhancement particularly shines is in cancer recovery patients. In a 2020 study, colorectal patients given Ginseng for 16 weeks had significant improvements in mood, enjoyment of life, and walking ability versus a placebo group.[4]

Given the power of Ginseng to resist fatigue and support energy production, it may be tempting to bring it into your daily routine. Yet the modern American is typically not the ideal candidate for Ginseng. People who are already overstimulated, fueled by excessive caffeine, and driven to their limits may find Ginseng pushes them over the edge. The energizing effects of Ginseng can mask the underlying symptoms of depletion. Therefore, it's key to address nutrition, sleep, and any underlying conditions while using Ginseng. While it's still a real Adaptogen, it's important to keep balance in mind when stretched thin or when sick. For slightly cooler and milder effects, it's important to know that Ginseng has an American sister, American Ginseng (*Panax quinquefolius*), a species with closely related functional benefits native to eastern North America. It may be a better place to start if you have a fiery, hot, pitta, energetic, or type-A personality.

HELPFUL WITH LIBIDO

Ginseng has been used as an aphrodisiac for thousands of years. Research shows it can speed up the development of reproductive organs and improve overall sexual performance.[5] In a randomized, placebo-controlled, double-blind study, patients with diagnosed erectile dysfunction who took 900 milligrams of Ginseng three times per day for eight weeks had improved sexual desire, intercourse satisfaction, and significant improvement in erectile dysfunction versus the placebo group.[6]

The libido benefits of Ginseng are also applicable for women, specifically during menopause. In a randomized, placebo-controlled, double-blind study, menopausal women took three grams of Ginseng per day divided into three doses of one gram each, and most had improved sexual arousal.[7]

HELPFUL WITH BRAIN

The main active constituents in Ginseng are ginsenosides, which have been shown to increase neurotransmitter activity and blood flow to the brain. A randomized, placebo-controlled, double-blind study out of Denmark found that individuals over the age of 40 who were given 400 milligrams of standardized Ginseng extract for eight weeks showed faster reactions and significant improvement in abstract thinking versus the placebo group.[8]

In another randomized, placebo-controlled, double-blind study put on by a human cognitive neuroscience unit, young individuals who took 400 milligrams of Ginseng per day showed improved secondary memory performance, speed of performing memory tasks, and accuracy of attentional tasks versus the placebo group.[9]

PREPARATION, SOURCING, AND DOSAGE

In many of its native regions, wild Ginseng is either endangered or extinct. Luckily, farmers began to cultivate Ginseng, and they became the source of the Ginseng commonly used today in TCM and distributed globally. Yet beware of "gas station" products that particularly call out Ginseng for libido effects. Quality and proper dosing are key to ensure you are getting the real deal and in turn, receiving Ginseng's benefits.

There are a few things to look out for when buying Ginseng in the marketplace. Even if you are purchasing the *Panax Ginseng* species, there are different colors of the root to be aware of: red, white, and black. Red Ginseng is unpeeled, steamed, and then dried before going to market. This is the most traditional way to prepare and use Ginseng in TCM. White Ginseng is also unpeeled but has not been steamed. It gets directly dried and then sold. The newest type of Ginseng on the market is black Ginseng. It is developed from a new method where the root is steamed and dried multiple times before being sold.

Red and white Ginseng are the types you will most likely see in the market, usually as a whole dried root, tincture, liquid extract, powder, or capsule. Red Ginseng is more warming, and white Ginseng is more cooling, so we suggest choosing the variety most appropriate for your body type (if you are cooler in constitution, choose red; if warmer, consider white).

If using the whole Ginseng root, ask the supplier or grower about the age of the root. This can be a distinguishing factor in quality. A good indicator of age is how "ugly" the root looks. Older roots have had more bugs and insects try to eat them, which makes them create more protective compounds that are also beneficial for humans. Older roots tend to be more bitter, which increases their medicinal potency (bitter = better).

An effective dose of the dry root ranges from 0.5 gram to 4.5 grams. If using the dry root, we suggest two to three grams per day as a strong but effective starting dose. This can be directly chewed or decocted. If decocting, bring about one quart of water to a boil and add the two to three grams of chopped Ginseng root. Let simmer for a minimum of 20 minutes and then drink throughout the day.

If using a standardized extract, start with 200 mg per day. This can be taken all at once or broken up into two dosages in the morning and midafternoon. You can build up to 400 milligrams per day if needed after slowly increasing by about 50 milligrams at a time every few days.

Starting small is always recommended, especially when it comes to Ginseng. Research shows that while it is safe to take Ginseng long-term, it's best to take it for 2 to 12 weeks and then take a break.[10] This is because Ginseng can be so powerfully energizing that it has the potential to mask underlying symptoms if those are not simultaneously being treated or supported. Taking a break will allow you to assess how your body has adjusted with the support of Ginseng before deciding to continue, or perhaps you may have reached your desired intention with taking it and no longer need its support.

REAL-LIFE WAYS TO BENEFIT FROM GINSENG

- *For energy:* Take as a daily decocted tonic for elderly people for a lift in energy and stamina, and to help combat weakness.

- *For libido:* Chew on the root to increase energy in menopausal women or to increase libido in an exhausted state.

- *For brain:* Use sparingly as a powder added to smoothies to increase cognition.

CORDYCEPS

Full legal name: *Cordyceps sinensis* and *Cordyceps militaris* from the *Ascomycete* parasite clan

Nicknames: Himalayan Viagra, Cordy-sex, caterpillar fungus

Power hub: Mushroom fruiting body

Home: Born in the Himalayan mountains. Loves being above 13,000 feet. Has been spotted in Nepal, India, China, and Tibet. Rare and unsustainable in the wild.

Energetics: Warm, moist

Helpful with:

1. Energy
2. Endurance
3. Libido

Comes with:

- Cordycepic acid, aka D-mannitol
- Cordycepin
- Adenosine
- Polysaccharides[11]

Common uses: Pre- and post-workout and high-altitude adventures

Best friends: Schisandra, Cacao, mint, rose hips, and ginger

Note: There are over 400 species of Cordyceps, all with unique characteristics, but most of the history is likely to be with Ophiocordyceps sinensis. We now use and recommend its close cousin Cordyceps militaris because it's scalable, sustainable, plant-based/vegan, ethical, and equally, if not more medicinal, than the unsustainable Ophiocordyceps sinensis.

A BRIEF HISTORY: From Horny Yaks to Professional Athletes

For over 2,000 years, Himalayan dwellers have searched the mountains for Cordyceps. They were originally discovered by Sherpas, who would herd their yaks in the high elevation mountainside in early spring. When they'd climb above 13,000 feet in elevation, they noticed their yaks would find and consume little mushrooms. Shortly after consuming them, they would go into heat, jumping in sexual excitement. This behavior ignited the Sherpas to try the mushroom for themselves and they noticed similar results. They felt improved stamina, had an increase in libido, and had an easier time breathing at these high elevations.

The Sherpas brought the mushroom to monks in their village, and its reputation spread from there. Eventually, word got to the emperor of China's physician, who prescribed it for the emperor. The effects were so great that a law was put into place that any Cordyceps found across the country must be brought directly to the emperor!

In the early 18th century, a French Jesuit priest, Perennin Jean-Baptiste Du Halde, was invited to be a guest at the emperor's court in China. Upon his stay, he became ill and was introduced to Cordyceps as a suggested ally to support his recovery. He was amazed by the effectiveness and declared it was worth four times its weight in silver! He brought back several mushrooms with him to France and published his account of Cordyceps, which spread to the scientific community, even leading to the discovery of using microorganisms to control crop pests. It was said that the mushroom made its debut in the U.S. in the mid-nineteenth century when Chinese immigrants building railroads used Cordyceps to support their lungs and immune system, and were not afflicted by the ailments of other builders.[12,13]

Cordyceps' reputation became noteworthy to the rest of the world after the 1993 World Championships in Athletics in Stuttgart, Germany. China's female running team won six of the nine possible medals in long-distance track and field. Rumors spread about the women doping or using illegal substances to achieve such impressive times, but no illegal activity was discovered. Ma Junren, the Chinese coach, however, said he had included Cordyceps in their protocol. As a legal and effective performance enhancer, Cordyceps' popularity quickly spread among professional athletes.

HELPFUL WITH ENERGY

Cordyceps has been used to support energy, from athletes to the elderly, for thousands of years. It's known to combat fatigue, invigorating your body without stimulation. Whenever people don't believe in the power of functional mushrooms, we like to give them a 1.5 gram dose of extracted Cordyceps fruiting body. It's one of the few natural medicines that can be felt within about 20 to 30 minutes of ingesting. Most report feeling a lift in energy and a heightened sense of physical awareness.

It's a powerful pre-workout mushroom because you can see a noticeable improvement in performance. But we never want to *rely* on anything to reach our performance goals or feel optimal. All Adaptogens should be used in addition to building a strong foundation through proper diet, exercise, and sleep. So, to reap long-term benefits from Cordyceps, we recommend taking post-workout, in recovery.

In a randomized double-blind, placebo-controlled clinical trial published in the *Chinese Journal of Integrative Medicine*, the VO_2 max (maximum oxygen uptake) of elderly volunteers who took three grams of Cordyceps per day for six weeks was significantly increased, while the placebo had no effect.[14]

In another study, mice who received low, medium, and high doses (40, 80, and 160 milligrams per kilogram per day) of *Cordyceps militaris* for 28 days showed that Cordyceps significantly postponed exhaustion in a swimming test and decreased concentrations of serum lactic acid, confirming the anti-fatigue and fatigue-resistance effects of *Cordyceps militaris*.[15] We often recommend Cordyceps for athletes, the elderly, and people who are chronically tired. It can also be helpful with people who have trouble breathing (for example, those with asthma).

HELPFUL WITH ENDURANCE

A major part of endurance is the ability to maintain a steady heart rate. Cardiac health and endurance go hand in hand. The opposite of a steady and strong heartbeat is known as cardiac arrhythmia, a disturbed or abnormal heartbeat that can lead to strokes. Many studies have been done on the use of Cordyceps to support cardiac health, showing partial and complete recoveries from arrythmia with the help of Cordyceps. In a clinical trial at Guangzhou Medical University in China, over 80 percent of the group who took 1.5 grams of Cordyceps per day showed cardiac improvement over a placebo group.[16]

Cordyceps improves the function of our HPA axis, the system in our body reacting to stress. By calming the HPA, our entire nervous system can relax. In a double-blind, placebo-controlled trial at UCLA School of Medicine, individuals who took Cordyceps showed increased oxygen intake from 1.88 to 2.00 liters per minute,[17] confirming how Cordyceps can improve exercise capacity and resistance to fatigue.

In Danielle's private practice, she would often formulate with Cordyceps for high-performance athletes to help with post-exercise recovery and increased long-term stamina.

HELPFUL WITH LIBIDO

From infertility to sexual dysfunction, this mushroom is a go-to for libido, causing it to gain nicknames like Cordy-sex and Himalayan Viagra. It has been used particularly for male sexual hypofunction, but it supports female libido as well. Positive studies have been done with Cordyceps in conjunction with IVF for fertility.[18] The positive effects are likely due to its ability to stimulate estradiol production.

In one study that examined cordycepin, an active constituent in Cordyceps, the results showed that Cordyceps had immense therapeutic value in fighting age-related male sexual dysfunctions.[19]

An interesting study done with boars examined Cordyceps' spermatogenic effect. The boars were given Cordyceps for two months, and their semen was collected and analyzed once per week. The quality and quantity of fertile sperm was significantly enhanced after one month, peaked in the second month, and had benefits that lasted for two weeks post-treatment. In addition, percentages of motile sperm cells and sperm motility improved significantly in the Cordyceps group, showing that Cordyceps may be of support with sexual enhancement.[20]

PREPARATION, SOURCING, AND DOSAGE

Sourcing is very important when it comes to Cordyceps. There are about 600 species of Cordyceps that have been identified worldwide. Most clinical research is on *Cordyceps sinensis, Cordyceps militaris* and a strain cultivated by Chinese mycologists in the 1960s called CS-4.

Cordyceps sinensis harvested in the wild is highly concerning. Due to its high value and rarity, there has been extensive overharvesting and poaching. Today, Cordyceps is extremely rare in the wild. The environmental and humanitarian concerns here are critical, which is why we suggest always buying cultivated Cordyceps strains, not wild varieties. This shouldn't be hard to do, as most wild strains will either be outrageously expensive or not the real thing. Luckily, cultivated varieties of Cordyceps have also been shown to have very similar benefits to the wild strains. Cultivated Cordyceps are also verified vegan, whereas the wild ones are a mix between the fungi and what it grew from, which is often various insect species.

As with all functional mushrooms, look for the extracted fruiting bodies (never raw or myceliated grain). While we usually caution against using mushrooms grown on grain for human consumption, Cordyceps is an exception. All other functional mushrooms discussed in this book are naturally found on wood. Our beloved little Cordyceps is not. Yet, it's still important to avoid the starches and fillers common in laboratory-grown mycelium products. One way to avoid this is to buy Cordyceps that has been grown in a myceliated liquid culture. The most common liquid culture–grown strain is the *CS-4 Cordyceps*, although we still prefer *Cordyceps militaris* for most health benefits as it has a Cordyceps fruiting body that is closer to its wild ancestors.

REAL-LIFE WAYS TO BENEFIT FROM CORDYCEPS

- *For energy:* Take if exhausted or depleted for a boost in physical energy. Or add a scoop of extracted powder to a warm beverage when heading to high-altitude places or mountainous regions, where oxygen is lower.

- *For endurance:* Drink a decocted tea or add a scoop of extracted powder to a smoothie in the recovery period of athletic training.

- *For libido:* Drink about 30 to 60 minutes before heading into the bedroom with a lover.

Perform *(Energy and Performance)* Case Study

When living in Colorado at high elevation, Danielle would often lean on Cordyceps. It was particularly helpful when her family living at sea level in California would come to visit. She would take them up the mountains to hike around her house shortly after their arrival. When the altitude passed around 8,000 feet, they would be huffing and puffing up the mountain. The thin air from the altitude change was immediately noticeable and caused a much more challenging hike. When they accepted her offer of a cup of tea made from Cordyceps mushroom extract before the hike, they cruised up the hills with surprising ease compared to without it. The increase in VO_2 max resulted in an almost immediate ability to breathe and move at higher altitudes with more ease and greater endurance.

MACA

Full legal name: *Lepidium meyenii* from the *Brassicaceae* family (just like all cruciferous veggies)

Nicknames: Nature's Viagra, pepper weed, Peruvian Ginseng (note: it is not a real Ginseng)

Power hub: Root, but it's technically a hypocotyl (a vegetable related to mustard, cauliflower, broccoli, and brussels sprouts)

Home: High up in the Peruvian Andes

Energetics: Warm, moist

Helpful with:

1. Energy
2. Libido
3. Stress

Comes with:

- Essential amino acids
- Fatty acids (linoleic acid, palmitic acid, and oleic acids)
- Phytosterols (sitosterol, campesterol, ergosterol, and brassicasterol)
- Minerals: potassium, calcium, phosphorus, iron, manganese, copper, zinc, sodium, iodine, bismuth, tin
- Saponins and tannins
- Macaenes and macamides
- Vitamins C, B1, B2, and B6

Common uses: All kinds of movement, particularly foreplay

Best friends: Cacao, Goji, probiotics, digestive enzymes, hemp seeds, and coconut oil

A BRIEF HISTORY: The Root to Get It On

From Spanish conquerors and Inca warriors to people of high mountain climates, Maca has a long tradition of being a powerhouse food for those who need strength and stamina. Maca is packed with nutrients, containing about 10 percent protein, 59 percent carbohydrates, and more fatty acids than any other root crop. Its use dates back to 1400 B.C. and it has been actively cultivated in the Peruvian mountains for 1,600 years. As the highest elevation food crop in the world, Maca thrives at altitudes between 10,000 and 15,000 feet in the Andean mountains. Despite being faced with 50-degree daily temperature changes, violent winds, and poor rocky soils, this strong root is adaptable and resilient. These are also qualities we can gain from consuming Maca.

While the oral legend is older than textual evidence, it was first written about in a 1553 chronicle of the Spanish conquest of the Andes. Legends tell of Inca warriors consuming plentiful amounts of the root before going to battle to improve their powers. Later, Spanish conquerors fed Maca to their cows to help them with high altitude sickness.

Maca is a root that represents power—in battle and in bed. It has been valued so highly that it's even been used as a currency.

HELPFUL WITH ENERGY

Maca has a long-held reputation as a caffeine-free energy booster. It provides energy without taxing the adrenals, leading to sustained energy without a crash, and is used to help with improving endurance, blood oxygenation, and muscle-building. There's even a playful term coined "Maca butt" used by women who take Maca alongside targeted exercise for the booty building benefits!

In one study, trained cyclists were divided into two groups, one that took Maca and the other a placebo. The cyclists completed a timed 40-kilometer trial before supplementing with Maca. They then took Maca (or a placebo) for 14 days. The same

40-kilometer ride was completed and timed. Those who took Maca significantly improved their cycling performance compared to the baseline test.[21]

HELPFUL WITH LIBIDO

Maca is perhaps most well known for its libido-supportive qualities in both men and women. As a nutritive tonic, it has been shown to support vitality and sexual function and can help stabilize hormone activity, treat impotence, ease menopausal troubles, and boost sperm count.[22] It has a unique ability to support libido. Instead of targeting just the sexual organs, it has a whole-body effect, including targeting hormonal imbalance and mood.[23]

There are several constituents linked to Maca's range of libido-enhancing effects. Maca contains arginine, a substance clinically linked to increased semen production.[24] Its sterols lend to its sex-enhancing effects, and its macamides and macaenes contribute to general energy enhancement.[25] There have been several human and animal trials proving Maca's ability to improve semen quality,[26] raise hormone levels in healthy adult men,[27] and increase sexual stamina.

A randomized, double-blind, placebo-controlled trial testing Maca's effect on men with mild erectile dysfunction found that the group taking 2.4 grams of Maca extract for 12 weeks showed more improvement in ED and experienced significant improvement in sexual performance.[28]

Another study sought to determine whether Maca was effective for selective-serotonin reuptake inhibitor (SSRI)–induced sexual dysfunction. This trial was conducted by the Depression Clinical and Research Program of the Department of Psychiatry at Massachusetts General Hospital. Patients with SSRI-induced sexual dysfunction were given either a low (1.5 grams per day) or high (3 grams per day) dose of Maca. The patients taking the higher dose had significant improvement in their scores, while the lower dose patients did not. The patients taking Maca also had significantly improved libido.[29]

HELPFUL WITH STRESS

While packed with amino acids, vitamins, and minerals, Maca's stress- and hormone-balancing effects are thought to be due to two unique phytonutrients, macaenes and macamides.[30] As a whole, Maca stimulates all glands in the HPA axis. This supports your body's ability to tolerate stressors and return to a state of equilibrium.

As Adaptogens often do, improvement in one bodily function leads to improvements elsewhere. Although the excitement around Maca is (understandably) in the energy and libido arena, these benefits also help improve our body's ability to handle stress. It's very common that new Maca users initially report more stimulative benefits. Yet with continued use, their bodies achieve balance (homeostasis), and the Maca eventually has a calming effect. It's a perfect example of the two-directional power of Adaptogens.

PREPARATION, SOURCING, AND DOSAGE

Maca is usually sold as an extracted powder or capsule but can sometimes be found as the whole cut and dried root. Most commonly, the root is harvested, dried, and then quickly ground into a powder to best preserve it. A powdered Maca can stay potent ("good") for up to seven years. After that, if properly stored, it won't necessarily spoil but will lose potency the longer it sits. It's best to store Maca powder in a dark amber bottle (we recommend Miron glass) in a cool place (cupboard or the refrigerator) out of direct sunlight.

There are eight varieties of Maca, each with a slightly different phytochemical profile. The types most commonly available are yellow, red, or black. Most people prefer yellow due to its slightly sweeter flavor. Over 30 percent of the Maca on the market is dried and powdered yellow root. However, the quality of Maca should be assessed by smell and taste rather than color. Good quality Maca should have a strong and *heavy* smell, with a bold, slightly pungent flavor. Ideally, the Maca is sourced from its natural environment, high in the Peruvian Andes, and harvested at maturity. However, there have recently been cases of over-harvesting and even stealing Maca from the Andes and bringing it into China. As such, try to purchase Maca and other Adaptogens from brands that disclose their sourcing to ensure the highest ethical and sustainable practices possible.

If using a powder, a good starting dose is one gram per day. If you are sensitive, you can divide the serving into two to three separate doses and space them out throughout the day. Once you've gotten used to the one gram dosage, you can slowly build up to about three grams. This might happen in a few days or over multiple weeks. Some people experience gas with Maca (as is common with some tubers). If this is the case, try taking it with digestive-supporting herbs or supplements such as probiotics, enzymes, or Goji.

REAL-LIFE WAYS TO BENEFIT FROM MACA

- *For energy:* Add to a morning smoothie for an extra boost of energy or mix into tea or coffee in the morning or midday for a pick-me-up.

- *For stress:* Add a scoop into homemade raw chocolate and break off a piece to keep stress at bay.

- *For libido:* Ditch the Viagra and try a scoop of Maca instead.

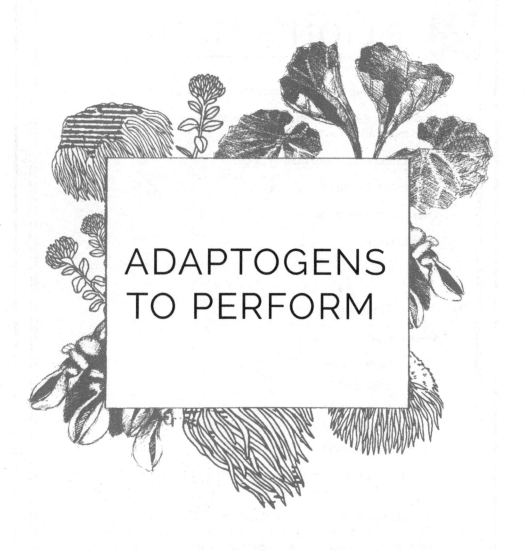

ADAPTOGENS TO PERFORM

FOR BRAIN AND FOCUS

LION'S MANE

Full legal name: *Hericium erinaceus* from the house of Russula

Nicknames: Pom-pom mushroom, hedgehog mushroom, monkey's head mushroom, Yamabushitake

Power hub: Mushroom fruiting body

Home: Asia and North America

Energetics: Neutral, neutral

Helpful with:

1. Brain
2. Longevity
3. Immunity

Comes with:

- Hericenones
- Erinacines
- Beta-d-glucans
- Hericium erinaceus polysaccharide
- Polypeptides

Common uses: To help you power through any sluggish afternoons when your brain is tapping out

Best friends: Cacao, Mucuna, Rhodiola, vitamin C, niacin (vitamin B3), coffee, caffeine (in natural, whole-food sources like guayusa, yerba mate, or green tea), and psilocybin containing mushrooms

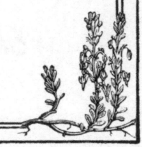

A BRIEF HISTORY: From Native American Tribes to Michelin Star Restaurants

A bright white mushroom with strands of cascading hairs, Lion's Mane is our favorite fungi for focus. And no, it does not have anything to do with the mane of a lion, apart from its captivating appearance. From Asia to North America, Lion's Mane has been harvested, extracted, and used as both a food and medicine for millennia. Stories are told of Native American tribes carrying this mushroom in their medicine bags to use as a styptic (a substance that stops bleeding). On the other side of the world, Lion's Mane was referred to as Yamabushitake, after the hermit Zen Japanese Yamabushi mountain monks. Maybe because they liked consuming Lion's Mane tea with meditation? In Traditional Chinese Medicine, it's prescribed for digestive issues like ulcers and gastritis. In Scandinavia, the mushroom is used to support the immune system in cancer patients. And worldwide, it is also a culinary treat that has been featured on the menus of Michelin star restaurants due to its incredible resemblance in taste and texture to crab and lobster meat. (You must try Lion's Mane sauteed with butter and a pinch of salt!)

HELPFUL FOR THE BRAIN

Known as the *smart mushroom*, Lion's Mane has proven abilities to support our cognition and brain. For example, in one "gold standard" study out of Nagano, Japan, 50- to 80-year-old men and women with mild cognitive impairment either took 250 milligrams of Lion's Mane three times per day for 16 weeks or a placebo.[1] The people taking Lion's Mane had significant improved cognitive function versus the placebo group. They also had better cognitive function each week while consuming the mushroom, but the study continued beyond the dosing to assess aftereffects and it revealed that cognitive benefits started to decline again after they stopped consuming it.

The two primary active brain compounds in Lion's Mane are *hericenones* and *erinacines*. *Hericenones* can help our brain produce more of a protein called nerve growth factors (NGF) that is produced in our hippocampus and regenerates neurons in our brain. NGF was discovered in the 1950s by two faculty members at Washington University in St Louis. They eventually won a Nobel Prize for this discovery in the late 1980s, but NGF is still a relatively new concept in the world of health.

While Astragalus and supplements like vitamin D, zinc, and melatonin could potentially support NGF, Lion's Mane is one of the only natural foods that has been proven to help produce it. As such, it's often touted as one of the safest and best "smart drugs," also called nootropics, and it is nature's best-known tool for neuroplasticity—the brain's ability to form and reorganize synaptic connections. This is especially valuable for learning new things.

HELPFUL FOR LONGEVITY

Erinacines, the other main constituent in Lion's Mane, have the rare ability to penetrate the blood-brain barrier. Other things that can cross this barrier are alcohol, nicotine, heroin, and caffeine, making erinacines look like a real saint.

To protect itself, the brain has a barrier that very few things can pass through. Good news for safety but bad news for delivering the brain with the supportive nutrients it needs. This impacts longevity because changes in brain chemistry can begin up to 20 to 30 years *before* signs of dementia begin.

Together with hericenones, erinacines help to support our brain's longevity. Simply put, a decrease in NGF leads to brain cells dying faster, weaker memory, and declining neuroplasticity. All bad things for longevity. And this is not just a matter of the longevity of our memory. Lion's Mane has a positive effect on nerves in other areas of your body as well.

In a study from Malaysia, researchers gave Lion's Mane extract to rats with damaged gluteal nerves (important nerves of the buttocks). After consuming the mushroom, the rats recovered so profoundly that they were able to walk again.[2] Given that most brain and nervous system research has been done in the last few decades, there's a limited number of human studies on anything, but promising research on Lion's Mane's benefits for neurodegenerative diseases like Parkinson's and Alzheimer's is starting to happen.[3] There's even early evidence that erinacines could help with mood and pain tolerance.

HELPFUL FOR IMMUNITY

Just like many other top mushrooms, Lion's Mane contains polysaccharides beneficial for our health. These complex (poly) sugars (saccharides) have two main benefits: they support gut health and are immunomodulatory. This means they act like "cruise control" for the immune system, ensuring it is neither too passive nor overactive. The most powerful and well-studied of these polysaccharides are beta-glucans, a common compound found in all top functional mushrooms. Lion's Mane also has its own unique polysaccharide called HEP (*Hericium erinaceus* polysaccharide), which has been shown to help balance or modulate our immune response by enhancing natural killer cells and macrophage activity. It regulates these cells in the immune system pathways of our intestines. Targeting the immune system via the gut, where about 70 percent of immune cells can be found, is a common theme among functional mushrooms. Basically, strong gut health equals a strong immune system, and vice versa.

Beyond the polysaccharides, the same constituents that support the brain may also play an important role in the health of the immune system. The way that NGF interacts with the immune system can most notably be seen after an injury, where levels of NGF are often increased. You might have experienced this the last time you had the flu, where your brain seemed to work poorly, and your nervous system followed. Similarly to how we have a strong gut-brain connection, we also have a brain-immunity connection.

PREPARATION, SOURCING, AND DOSAGE

Lion's Mane is most commonly available in extracted powders. This extraction—usually done with hot water—helps unlock its active water-soluble compounds. Be wary of words like fermented, micronized, or powdered. Always seek out the word extraction on packaging (or extract it yourself) for the highest absorption in your body. If the mushroom is not extracted, your body will not be able to utilize many of the beneficial compounds in the fruiting body.

The most common extracts are in a 10:1 ratio, but this may vary depending on the type and technique of extraction. For example, dual extraction is more valuable than just hot water extraction. And just like animals in nature and our ancestors did, always use the mushroom fruiting body. Studies show that the fruiting bodies contain 10 to 30 times the number of polysaccharides as mycelium.

Ideally, we would use wildcrafted Lion's Mane, but organically grown fruiting bodies are as good. Avoid lab-grown mycelium products and conventional (nonorganic) Lion's Mane due to their ability to collect heavy metals and toxins.

The most common daily dosage is 500 milligrams per day of properly extracted Lion's Mane fruiting body. This can be taken either all at once or 250 milligrams twice per day. You can increase the daily dosage to 1.5 grams for more noticeable and immediate results. In our experience, benefits plateau around three to five grams per day. The highest dose we have seen benefits with, even as a temporary solution post-surgery and for nerve pain, is five grams per day. However, you can increase effectiveness by pairing it with other vitamins or herbs. Any natural source of caffeine (coffee, green tea, guayusa), vitamin C, and niacin can help in delivery, which means you can take less and experience equal or greater benefits than higher doses alone.

REAL-LIFE WAYS TO BENEFIT FROM LION'S MANE

- *For brain:* Mix the powder into morning coffee or tea to get your brain going.

- *For longevity:* Mix into beverages or smoothies daily.

- *For immunity:* Add to soups or stews during the change of seasons or anytime you feel the sniffles coming on.

Perform *(Brain and Focus)* Case Study

Born with kyphosis and scoliosis, a woman who had chronic pain and back problems her whole life had corrective spinal fusion surgery to fuse her entire spine to two metal rods with 28 screws. She was told she would have pain for the rest of her life; it was just a matter of how intense it would be. After the surgery, she started doing physical therapy to learn to walk again. In the midst of her healing, she discovered Lion's Mane mushroom. Since then, she has taken it daily for over a year, and her recovery has gone faster than expected. To this day, she has no nerve damage aside from some superficial areas of numbness. Doctors were very surprised by how well and how quickly she healed. She attributes this in large part to the Lion's Mane and notes that beyond the physical and nerve healing benefits, she has more mental clarity, gets sick less often, and overall has less back pain.

MUCUNA

Full legal name: *Mucuna pruriens* from the *Fabaceae*, the legume and pea family

Nicknames: Velvet bean, monkey tamarind, cow-itch plant, kapikacchu, dopamine bean

Power hub: Fruit, but it's often also called a pod, seed, or bean

Home: India, Africa, tropical Asia, and the Caribbean

Energetics: Hot, neutral

Helpful with:

1. Brain
2. Libido
3. Stress

Comes with:

- Levodopa (aka L-dopa)
- Antioxidants
- Polyphenols
- Amino acids
- Glutathione, lecithin, gallic acid, beta-sitosterol

Common uses: Lifting you up when you're feeling down

Best friends: Ashwagandha, Gotu Kola, Maca, Lion's Mane, Cacao, green tea, L-theanine, coffee, and coconut

A BRIEF HISTORY: The Bean that Turns It All On

The magic velvet bean, Mucuna, is a natural nootropic ("smart drug") that's been used in Ayurveda and West Africa for centuries. The Mucuna vine grows abundantly across India and has been used for over two thousand years. Easy to spot in nature, it has long seed pods with a velvet coating of hairs (trichomes). These can irritate the skin and cause itching, which is why it has common names like kapikacchu, meaning "one starts itching like a monkey."

Part of the *Fabaceae* family, it's a legume along with common vegetables like peas and beans. The seed pod is the most commonly used part of the plant due to the amazing discovery of its L-dopa content, which is a natural cognitive and sexual performance enhancer. Yet beyond the fruit or seed pod, the root, trichomes (hairs on the seed pod), flowers, and leaves are also edible or medicinal.

In Central America and Africa, the leaves are highly revered. They're both eaten for nourishment and used medically. Folk uses range from treating bone fractures, dog bites, and ringworm, to scorpion stings, sores, and even syphilis. The seeds are also medicinal, with compounds that inhibit snake venom.[4] In Nigeria, the seeds are commonly used as a protein source in human and animal diets. In West Africa, the flowers are used for snake bites and as uterine stimulants (just what it sounds like, these are substances that increase the tone of the muscles of the uterus). In India, the bean is used as an aphrodisiac, neuroprotectant, and Adaptogenic tonic.

Mucuna is a tridoshic herb, meaning it balances all three of the doshas (or body types) in Ayurveda and therefore is a choice option to help harmonize all types of people. As part of the pea family, it's also quite nourishing, used to repair your body in times of depletion. It's ability to support the nervous, reproductive, and digestive systems make Mucuna a true Adaptogen to balance and restore the entire system.

HELPFUL WITH THE BRAIN

Mucuna seed is true brain food. It's best known for its main phenolic compound, levodopa or L-dopa. This amino acid plays an important role in mood, sex, and movement. When it comes to the brain, L-dopa acts as a precursor to the "feel-good" neurotransmitter dopamine. Insufficient amounts of dopamine contribute to depression, while excess levels can lead to mania. Thus, a balanced supply of dopamine in the brain is critical. It helps maintain proper motor coordination, emotional health, a strong memory, and neuroendocrine regulation. The right amount of dopamine is key to a physically and mentally healthy brain. L-dopa also affects the neurotransmitter serotonin, which helps regulate our mood and feelings of well-being, and has been studied as an antidepressant. L-dopa is an effective regulator of healthy brain chemistry and elevated mood.

One of the symptoms of neurodegenerative diseases is a decline in dopamine-containing neurons. In advanced stages of Alzheimer's, Parkinson's, and dementia, this neuron decline can be up to 50 percent. While there are no "cures" for these diseases, L-dopa is often prescribed to help provide preventative and symptomatic relief from continued brain degradation.

Mucuna contains the natural form of L-dopa. Since your body recognizes whole foods better than isolates, Mucuna may be a safer and more effective option than pure, isolated L-dopa. When using the whole bean, many other phytochemicals work in concert with the natural L-dopa, producing greater benefit with fewer side effects compared to the conventional prescribed L-dopa. Mucuna's natural L-dopa has a quicker onset time, has a longer-lasting effect, and works better than isolated L-dopa due to the synergistic compounds in the seed that are not present with the isolated version. Early evidence also shows that the other compounds present in the seed may also have neuroprotective benefits.

Beyond L-dopa, Mucuna contains powerful antioxidants, most notably polyphenols. These, like all antioxidants, scavenge dangerous free radicals in your body. They can also cross the blood-brain barrier and exert antioxidant action on the brain, which supports brain longevity.

HELPFUL WITH LIBIDO

Mucuna has been used as a sex booster and tonic for reproductive purposes in both men and women for centuries. In Ayurvedic medicine, it is used for its support with infertility issues related to psychological distress. And with an affinity for the nervous system, Mucuna is both strengthening and calming.

For example, in a study conducted by the Department of Biochemistry at King George's Medical University in India, men suffering from psychological stress associated with infertility who were each given five grams per day of Mucuna seed powder for three months showed that treatment with Mucuna significantly reduced psychological stress and improved sperm count and motility. It also restored levels of critical antioxidant SOD, catalase, GSH, and ascorbic acid. It was concluded that Mucuna counteracts infertility through managing stress, reactivating the antioxidant defense system, and improving semen quality.[5]

Beyond infertility, Mucuna has been used as an overall sex tonic with impressive results in vivo, meaning in human or animal trials. It affects the HPA, which regulates reproduction, aging, and development. The boosting of brain hormones serotonin and dopamine also helps with mood and sex drive. The L-dopa directly increases dopamine in the brain and leads to increased libido, plasma testosterone, and activation of sexual behavior. Dopamine also triggers the increased synthesis of testosterone in the testes while simultaneously reducing mental stress. Mucuna essentially melts stress from the mind, allowing your body's energy to drop from brain to body and the vitality of the reproductive system to activate.

Many in vivo studies on the libido and aphrodisiac effects of Mucuna seed have shown Mucuna increases the frequency subjects have sex as well as their ejaculation latency. It successfully increases erections, recovers spermatogenic loss, and increases sperm count and sperm motility. Other studies have found it increases sexual desire, penile rigidity, erection, and duration of ejaculation with orgasm.[6] Time and time again, it has proven to be a powerful harmonizer of hormones, supporting the body on a physical, mental, and emotional level.

HELPFUL WITH STRESS

Like many of our Adaptogens, Mucuna is exposed to many stressors in nature. Its ability to thrive despite being faced with drought, low soil fertility, and high soil acidity lends to its ability to support our body in our fight against stress. Mucuna combats both cellular and emotional stress. Its antioxidants ameliorate oxidative stress on a neuronal and dermal level, and its L-dopa directly reduces stress by enhancing mood.

Mucuna is often used in individuals with Parkinson's disease, a condition that occurs when the nervous system progressively loses dopaminergic neurons and leads to problems with movement. Symptoms include resting tremors, rigidity, posture issues, and freezing. The disorder is thought to be at least in part related to oxidative stress. Mucuna's antioxidant action is critical to combating this oxidative stress.[7]

Oxidative stress from sun exposure (UV radiation), cigarette smoke, and daily toxins is extremely common today and requires the body to respond and combat toxic free radicals. Mucuna's antioxidant properties show promising potential for stress reduction, specifically targeted at skin-related pathologies like the above.

When it comes to battling stress, Mucuna is like a happiness bean. Its L-dopa activates dopamine, which has a powerful effect on mood and emotions. It regulates hormones that calm the nervous system and has an anti-anxiety and antidepressant effect. Beyond dopamine, Mucuna also activates other chemicals involved in moderating stress, such as serotonin and norepinephrine. Serotonin is responsible for modulating mood, learning, memory, sleep, and digestion. Norepinephrine is similar to adrenaline. It's an excitatory neurotransmitter that stimulates activity in the brain. It's also involved in regulating heart rate, blood pressure, alertness, memory, and arousal.

In one study, animals that were given Mucuna extract for two weeks exhibited an increase in serotonin and norepinephrine. As clinical studies show that depressed individuals don't have enough dopamine, norepinephrine, and serotonin, Mucuna's ability to activate all three of these crucial neurotransmitters means it's a powerful stress support and mood elevator.

PREPARATION, SOURCING, AND DOSAGE

Most commonly found in a powdered form, Mucuna can also be bought in a tincture, tablet, or capsules. We suggest beginning with 200 to 500 milligrams of Mucuna extract daily for one to two weeks. From there, increase the dose incrementally, stopping at five grams per day.

It's important to note that the dosage of pharmaceutical levodopa is not equivalent to L-dopa found in Mucuna. For example, 250 milligrams of Mucuna extract at 6 percent standardized L-dopa is equivalent to 15 milligrams of pure levodopa. As we previously discussed, when herbs are taken in their whole form, a synergistic effect takes place. This is especially true with Mucuna because it is so common to focus on the L-dopa in the bean. Yet it is critical to keep in mind that it is not just the L-dopa that has the benefit, but the combination of compounds that work with the L-dopa when ingested in its whole form that provide the most benefit.

REAL-LIFE WAYS TO BENEFIT FROM MUCUNA

- *For brain:* Add a scoop of powder into your morning cup of coffee for a brain-boosting preventative for neurodegenerative diseases, or to halt further neural degradation.

- *For libido:* Use as a daily fertility support for men or women trying to reproduce.

- *For stress:* Mix with Cacao and drink as a nourishing tonic to restore balance or mix into raw chocolate to elevate your mood.

GOTU KOLA

Full legal name: *Centella asiatica* from the *Apiaceae* family

Nicknames: Brahmi, Asian Pennywort

Power hub: Leaf

Home: Sri Lanka, Thailand, Vietnam, India, and the US—particularly Oregon and Florida in the spring

Energetics: Cool, moist

Helpful with:

1. Brain
2. Stress
3. Longevity

Comes with:

- Saponins
  - Well known:
    - Asiaticoside
    - Asiatic acid
    - Madecassoside
    - Centellasaponin
  - Newly discovered:
    - Centelloside
    - 11-oxo-asiaticoside/madecassoside
    - 11(β)-methoxy asiaticoside/madecassoside

Common uses: Art projects, study sessions, reading the morning paper

Best friends: Lion's Mane, bacopa, rosemary, peppermint, and spearmint

A BRIEF HISTORY: The Sacred Leaf of Creativity

Gotu Kola is part of the (infamous) *Apiaceae* (previously *Umbelliferae*) family. This family of herbs contains common culinary plants like cilantro and carrot, as well as deadly look-alikes including poison hemlock. Popular in both Traditional Chinese Medicine and Ayurveda, Gotu Kola is seen as a powerful medicine and spiritual tool.

Gotu Kola is often referred to by the Hindi name *Brahmi*, which translates to "creative forces of the earth." There are several herbs called Brahmi, so always reference the full Latin name to ensure you are getting Gotu Kola when looking to use this Adaptogenic leaf. In Ayurveda, it's a Rasayana, or general tonic, referred to as "a pharmacy in one herb." Over 2,000 years ago, it was recorded as a medicinal herb in the classic Chinese Shen-nong's Herbal Materia Medica. Since that time, it has been a prime tonic to promote mental clarity, calm the nervous system, and help with digestion. It's prescribed internally for syphilis, hepatitis, stomach ulcers, sore throats, diarrhea, fever, asthma, and UTIs. Today, it's used both internally and topically. Topically, its most common use is to help dissolve scar tissue, treat varicose veins, and heal wounds.

With the many uses of this sacred leaf, it is perhaps most well known as a nootropic: a true brain herb. Ever heard of the Doctrine of Signatures? Gotu Kola is a prime example of this concept. The leaf resembles a brain, so is thought to help balance the right and left hemispheres of the brain. And indeed, it does nourish the brain by improving concentration, increasing alertness, and helping your body cope with stress.

Fun fact: elephants, who are a symbol of longevity, are known to munch on Gotu Kola leaves!

The Doctrine of Signatures

The doctrine of signatures is the concept that how something looks in nature gives us an idea of how it supports our body. This doctrine is an ancient practice of observation of nature in which color, texture, shape, smell, and location all come into play. The observations are thought to be a poetic way of nature showing how plants and fungi may be supportive to humans. For example, a slice of a carrot looks like a human eye, therefore carrots must be good for eye health. Or walnuts look like a human brain and are thus supportive for brain health.

HELPFUL FOR THE BRAIN

Clearing brain fog and having a calm mental state is key to healthy mental function. Gotu Kola, another Ayurvedic Rasayana, is called a Medhya Rasayana, which is specific to being a brain tonic. It's been used to slow mental aging, regenerate neural tissues, and protect nerves. The daily benefits include enhanced memory, increased concentration, and improved creative thinking.[8]

Much of the neuroprotective and nootropic effects of Gotu Kola are thought to be due to triterpene compounds (asiatic acid, asiaticoside, and madecassoside). A second important group of compounds is caffeoylquinic acids, thought to have the potential to enhance the Nrf2-antioxidant response pathway.[9]

A study conducted in 2020 found a range of neuroprotective phytochemicals in alcohol extracts (tincture) of Gotu Kola. Beyond the original seven studied brain-supportive compounds in the leaf, six new compounds have recently been discovered. These new compounds are saponins, specifically glycosides,[10] molecules with a sugar bound to another functional group. They have been widely studied for their benefits to human health, including their role in inhibiting cancer cell proliferation.[11] The most neuroprotective compound in this group is 11-oxo-madecassoside, which activates an important pathway called the phosphatidylinositol 3-kinase/AKT pathway. Research has pointed to improvement of this important pathway's function contributing to brain recovery in stroke patients.[12] New research reveals how Gotu Kola supports the brain in more ways than previously understood. It also opens the door for researchers to continue to study this miraculous plant for its ability to protect and revive neurological function in all individuals.

HELPFUL WITH STRESS

A double-blind, placebo-controlled study assessed Gotu Kola's anxiolytic (anti-anxiety and stress-supportive) effects by evaluating the acoustic startle response (ASR) in humans. Subjects were either given a single 12-gram dose of Gotu Kola or a placebo. Results showed that Gotu Kola significantly attenuated the peak ASR amplitude 30 and 60 minutes post-treatment, confirming Gotu Kola's long-held applications in Ayurveda and TCM to relieve symptoms of anxiety.[13]

In another study, participants with generalized anxiety disorder (GAD) were given 500 milligrams two times per day for 60 days. Standard psychological questionnaires and stress rating scales taken at day 0 (baseline), day 30, and day 60 revealed that Gotu Kola significantly reduced stress and associated depression.[14] This is notable since there is only a limited pool of stress and anxiety-related studies on natural products, mostly because the modern concept of stress is relatively new.

HELPFUL FOR LONGEVITY

Energetically, Gotu Kola is thought to help develop the crown chakra, the seventh chakra located at the top of the head, which is one reason why yogis use it to assist in their meditation practice. This chakra is associated with higher states of consciousness, so strengthening it lends to a strong meditation practice, and a strong meditation practice is a key to longevity.

On a phytochemical level, Gotu Kola has antioxidants that help prevent age-related changes. These antioxidants impact the cortex, hypothalamus, striatum, cerebellum, and hippocampus of the brain. A study with rats put these anti-aging and longevity effects to the test. Rats given 300 milligrams per kilogram of their weight daily for 60 days showed positive improvements in all five examined brain regions compared to the control. The antioxidant potential also provides protection against age-related oxidative damage.[15]

Staying healthy and avoiding infections also contributes to a long and healthy life. Getting sick frequently takes a toll on your body. Thus, keeping your immune system strong directly correlates to longevity. Gotu Kola's triterpenoids have antimicrobial activities, protecting against infections.[16]

Lastly, and perhaps most interesting, is Gotu Kola's effect on telomerase. Telomerase activators are important for longevity and anti-aging. Without telomerase, cells will shorten and die. The shorter the telomeres, the quicker aging and age-related diseases occur. In an enlightening 2019 study, Gotu Kola was shown to increase telomerase activity nine-fold compared to no treatment.[17] This may be a key reason for Gotu Kola's anti-aging, cognitive, liver, and wound-healing benefits.

PREPARATION, SOURCING, AND DOSAGE

Gotu Kola is available in many forms, including as a dried herb, tincture, tablet, ointment, or capsules. Depending on the form, the suggested dose will vary. The dried herb is best made into an infusion. Simply pour one to two teaspoons of dried herb into a French press and cover with one cup boiling water. Let the infusion steep for about 20 minutes and then press. You can drink up to three cups per day. If using a tincture, look for a ratio of about 30 percent alcohol. We recommend using 30 to 60 drops up to three times per day. If using a standardized extract, start with 50 to 250 milligrams up to three times per day. Most studies are done with 90 to 120 milligrams daily in adults over the age of 18. If over 65, take a lower dose. Remember, you can always increase the dosage over time. It's safer for your body to start small and slowly build up from there as needed.

REAL-LIFE WAYS TO BENEFIT FROM GOTU KOLA

- *For brain:* Make an infusion and sip daily as a brain tonic.
- *For stress:* Add a scoop of powdered dried herb into a daily smoothie on days that stress and stakes are high.
- *For longevity:* Steep with mints and drink as a delicious daily tea for overall well-being day or night.

RHODIOLA

Full legal name: *Rhodiola rosea* from the *Crassulaceae* Family

Nicknames: Viking/golden/arctic/rose root, Nordic Ginseng (although not a real Ginseng)

Power hub: Root

Home: Cold climates, including Canada, Alaska, Mongolia, Russia, and Scandinavia

Energetics: Cool, dry

Helpful with:

1. Brain
2. Endurance
3. Stress

Comes with:

- Rosavins
- Salidrosides
- Flavonoids

Common uses: Helping you prepare for big adventures and long journeys

Best friends: Lion's Mane, Cacao, and slightly sweet things to balance its energetics, like honey

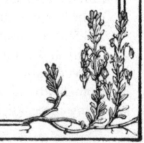

A BRIEF HISTORY: Marriage Bouquets to Viking Medicine

Rhodiola has a long history of use with the Vikings and people of Siberia. It's known to increase energy and keep the immune system strong during long, cold winters. In Nordic countries, indigenous Sami people chewed on the roots during arduous journeys to help with endurance. The Vikings took Rhodiola before going to battle. Inupiat natives from Alaska would use the flowers medicinally. This cooling and drying herb is a strengthener, both physically and energetically.

One of its common names is rose root. Some say this is because it has the scent of rose, but more fantastically, this name comes from its symbolic historical use. Newlyweds in the Siberian mountains were given a bouquet of Rhodiola on their wedding day. It was a symbol of fertility and healthy children to come.

The doctrine of signatures comes into play here again. (Reminder: this is when the nature of the plant gives us information about how it may affect the human body.) Rhodiola, like so many Adaptogens, is faced with extreme environmental adversities. When we were in Iceland in the summer of 2021, we found wild Rhodiola. It was growing in the most extreme places. Iceland's geography and climate are challenging enough. Yet Rhodiola took it to a new level. It wasn't just anywhere in the country. We found it hiding on the sides of cliff faces, in remote glacier zones, and among rough, rocky soil. From Iceland to Mongolia, it thrives in the most extreme climates on Earth. This ability to endure the elements transfers to the marriage analogy. Rhodiola gives newlyweds patience, strength, and endurance to persevere through the inevitable stressors of marriage. The folklore of these benefits is now confirmed by science. From legends to lab, this powerful little plant is one of the original and most studied Adaptogens.

This all-in-one root is neuro (brain), cardio (heart), hepatic (liver), and stress protective. From helping with mental and physical endurance to supporting hormones and fertility in men and women, Rhodiola's omnipotent benefits make it a favorite herb to many clinical herbalists.

HELPFUL FOR THE BRAIN

Multiple studies show Rhodiola extract has a protective effect on learning and memory. It enhances central nervous system activity and increases cognitive functions (attention, memory, etc.). It does this while also acting as a neuroenhancer that inhibits the aging of the brain. The first Materia Medica of Iceland said that Rhodiola "enhances the intellect," and the European Food Safety Authority (EFSA) praised Rhodiola as "contribut[ing] to optimal mental and cognitive activity." It is part of the official Russian pharmacopeia to this day as an antidepressant and nerve tonic.

A study published in *Phytomedicine* concluded that Rhodiola's effects were analogous to prescription drugs in reducing depression, with fewer side effects.[18]

The two main constituents in Rhodiola, rosavins and salidrosides, act as *neuroprotectants* that inhibit monoamine oxidase, which breaks down neurotransmitters. This way there are more neurotransmitters in the system (like dopamine and serotonin) for longer periods of time. These neurotransmitters are in part responsible for our mood, attention, and concentration.[19]

HELPFUL WITH ENDURANCE

Exercise is a form of stress on the body, particularly endurance exercise, which is physical activity that increases the heart rate and promotes increased use of oxygen in the body. Rhodiola's performance-enhancing and balancing effects shine in athletes. It reduces fatigue, treats symptoms of asthenia (loss of strength and energy) that come after intense physical exercise, and has an anti-fatigue action that works directly on muscles. It's thus used to treat stiffness and spasms after overworking and to restore weak nerves, particularly when you push your systems into exhaustion.

Fundamental to endurance is heart health. Several studies show Rhodiola's cardioprotective benefits, including helping to regulate an irregular heartbeat and protect against stress-induced heart disease. In addition, Rhodiola's antioxidants help protect the heart from stress-related damage.

A double-blind, placebo-controlled randomized study out of Belgium found that subjects given 200 milligrams of Rhodiola extract had increased breathing ability and took longer to get to an exhaustion phase compared to those who took the placebo, thus concluding that Rhodiola extract can improve endurance exercise performance.[20]

HELPFUL WITH STRESS

Rhodiola is the only Adaptogen for "stress" included in the Herbal Medicinal Products of the European Medicines Agency. This famously conservative committee is responsible for assessing scientific information on herbal medicines. Rhodiola is ". . . for temporary relief of symptoms of stress, such as fatigue and sensation of weakness."[21] It's rare that natural herbs or mushrooms are accepted in European countries as readily as Rhodiola is. Perhaps it's because it relieves symptoms of acute stress and prevents chronic stress, both things we all desperately need help with.

In a 2015 study out of the UK, participants who took 200 milligrams of Rhodiola two times per day over 14 days showed a significant reduction in stress, anger, confusion, and depression in self-reported cognitive tests.[22]

PREPARATION, SOURCING, AND DOSAGE

Rhodiola is sold as a tincture, capsules, powdered extract, or occasionally dried root. There are a few rules of thumb to ensure you are getting the highest quality and most efficacious product. If using a tincture, start with about 10 drops and work up to 30 drops after a few days. Once consistently at 30 drops (or one milliliter, aka one dropperful), you can increase the dose to 30 drops three times per day if needed. If you are into the DIY game and want to try making an extract yourself, make a decoction using one to two teaspoons of the dried root per every eight ounces of water. Decoct for a minimum of 20 minutes and up to several hours to increase strength and potency. Note that if you are drinking as a decoction, it can get quite astringent. If this happens, consider adding a corrigent like licorice or honey. The easiest way to consume it is in a capsule or powder, which you can add to smoothies, raw chocolate, or a cup of tea or coffee. Start with ¼ teaspoon of powder per day and build up to ½ teaspoon after a few days of consistent use.

REAL-LIFE WAYS TO BENEFIT FROM RHODIOLA

- *For brain:* Add powder into morning coffee to give your brain a boost.

- *For endurance:* Consume through the winter for endurance and physical strength despite the elements.

- *For stress:* Mix Rhodiola powder into raw chocolate and nibble on it in times of stress.

Morning Coffee Recipe for Brain and Performance

Try this powerful super coffee recipe anytime before noon. to crush your work tasks and to-do list without a crash later in the evening (note: the noon time limit is because of the caffeine, not because of the Adaptogens).

8 ounces of brewed organic coffee of your choice

1 teaspoon of Lion's Mane extract

1 teaspoon of Mucuna

1 teaspoon of Gotu Kola

1 tablespoon coconut oil

Splash of vanilla extract

Sprinkle of cinnamon powder

Sprinkle of cayenne powder

Hot foamed plant milk (optional)

Brew the coffee in your preferred way (coffee machine, pour-over, AeroPress, French press, etc.). Pour in a blender while still steaming hot with the oil and dry ingredients. Blend for 10 to 15 seconds and open carefully. Optionally, add hot foamed milk of your choice to make it a latte. Enjoy while hot!

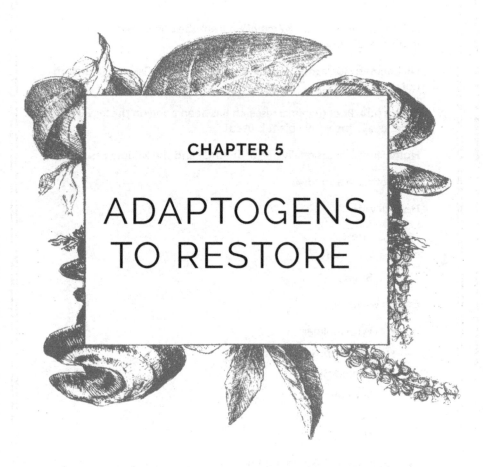

CHAPTER 5

ADAPTOGENS TO RESTORE

FOR STRESS AND MOOD

ASHWAGANDHA

Full legal name: *Withania somnifera* from the *Solanaceae* (nightshade) family

Nicknames: Horse root, winter/wild cherry, Indian Ginseng (although not a real Ginseng)

Power hub: Root (minimal research has been done on the leaves and occasionally the whole plant is used)

Home: India, occasionally in North Africa and the Middle East

Energetics: Warm, dry

Helpful with:

1. Stress
2. Longevity
3. Brain

Comes with:

- Withanolides
- Withaferins
- Sitoindosides
- Somniferine
- Iron
- Flavonoids

Common uses: Evening routines, especially that quiet time just before bed

Best friends: Adaptogens like Reishi, Tulsi, and Rhodiola, nut milk, ghee, honey, cinnamon, and cardamom

A BRIEF HISTORY: A Rasayana to Nourish and Revive

Ashwagandha is another Ayurvedic Rasayana. One of the most reputable plants in Ayurveda, its use dates back at least three thousand years and was used by common people and as a remedy of Hindu sages (Rishis) who were the personal physicians of the king. Its bright orange berries resemble tomatoes—a close relative to Ashwagandha—yet unlike tomato plants, the root holds its medicine. *Ashwa* means "horse" and *gandha* means "smell" in Sanskrit. The ground root famously smells a bit like a sweaty horse! It's believed that the root makes you as strong, calm, and graceful as a stallion. Although, when Danielle lived in India, she was told the horse association meant more than the smell.

Different from many other Adaptogens, Ashwagandha's Latin name *somnifera* means sleep-inducing. As a nourishing, restorative, and stress-supportive medicine, it can quicken the recovery time after illness, help you bounce back from extended stress, and calm the mind to prepare you for a restful sleep. It can also be paired with stimulants like coffee, to balance the effects of the caffeine.

Ashwagandha's uses stretch far beyond being calming and rejuvenating in Ayurveda. It has a strong association with women's health. It's used in parts of Africa as an indigenous medicine as an aphrodisiac and an abortifacient. In the West, it's a fertility tonic (but should not be taken during pregnancy, only in the months leading up to it). Because it's high in iron, antispasmodic, and relaxes the nervous system, it's also recommended for dysmenorrhea (painful periods) and to nourish breastfeeding mamas.

Beyond women's health, it's used in Africa to strengthen the immune system after fevers and inflammatory conditions. In Yemen, the dried leaves are used as a paste for wounds and burns as well as a natural sunscreen. The berries are used in various places around the world as a topical aid for tumors, carbuncles, and ulcers. Yet the root has carried on as the most potent and relevant part of the plant today. From treating anxiety and insomnia, aiding with muscle regeneration, and increasing production of HGH (human growth hormone) to aiding in respiratory health, supporting a healthy libido, and as a general tonic to female repro-duction, Ashwagandha has been proven to strengthen, soothe, and nourish many systems of your body.[1]

HELPFUL WITH STRESS

Ashwagandha supports the nervous system by promoting healthy levels of "the stress hormone" cortisol. A low and healthy amount of cortisol results in a calm, balanced mood, but when it's in excess, it can lead to anxiety. Cortisol should be highest in the morning, to help you pop out of bed with energy. Then, as the day goes on, it should slowly decrease. By the end of the day, cortisol should be at its lowest point, allowing you to get to sleep.

This ideal curve often gets interrupted by stress, which triggers additional cortisol. In a double-blind, placebo-controlled study, one group receiving 300 milligrams of Ashwagandha two times per day (a total of 600 milligrams per day) for 60 days had a sig-nificant reduction on all stress-assessment scales, including serum (blood) cortisol levels.[2] A second study of equally high standards showed that participants who took Ashwagandha had less cortisol, a lowered heart rate, and improved blood pressure—all without adverse effects—helping to reduce feelings of stress and anxiety.[3]

HELPFUL WITH LONGEVITY

Ashwagandha has long been used as a tonic for longevity. It was given to those whose nervous system was worn out, whether from old age or long-term stress. When the nervous system is depleted, a cascade of symptoms can arise. Ashwagandha effec-tively nourishes and revitalizes many organs of your body, from the liver to the thyroid.

Ashwagandha's antioxidants directly protect the liver, our body's largest internal organ. It's often pigeonholed as being the body's center for detoxification. Yet liver health is critical to over-all well-being since it also manages your body's blood sugar and urea cycle, removes bacteria from the bloodstream, and much more. Ashwagandha is right up there with other top liver herbs like milk thistle. In one animal study, rats that developed liver lesions from an insecticide were completely cured after 48 days of treatment with Ashwagandha root.[4] Another study showed that Ashwagandha's antioxidants protected the liver from the side effects of common medications. It's even been effective in treating NAFLD (nonalcoholic fatty liver disease), a disease that 10 to 25 percent of the global population is affected by. Ashwagandha can also help balance thyroid hormones.

HELPFUL FOR THE BRAIN

An ancient use of Ashwagandha was to boost memory and aid in intellect. Newer modern research shows that its regenerative properties can slow, stop, and even reverse damage to brain cells.[5] Other studies show its potential in reconstructing neural networks. Much of the brain-related research on Ashwagandha centers on a medication called KSM-66, which is essentially a concentration of Ashwagandha root's key medical phytochemicals. There's another branded Ashwagandha product called Sensoril, which also has strong clinical research.

Oxidative stress damages cells everywhere in your body, including the brain. Withanolides, perhaps the most studied compound present in Ashwagandha, are shown to protect nerve cells from oxidative damage. Research shows that withanolides may additionally prevent the formation of beta-amyloid fibrils,[6] a common component in the development of neurodegenerative diseases like Alzheimer's.

Ashwagandha has also been shown to protect nerve cells against toxic damage. In early in vitro studies, there are even signs of it promoting nerve cell growth, making it neuroprotective. This can be thought of as armor protecting the precious brain from toxic stressors.

In a randomized, double-blind, placebo-controlled trial, adults with mild cognitive impairment received Ashwagandha extract. These individuals were considered at high risk to develop neurodegenerative diseases later in life. The trial group was given 300 milligrams of KSM-66 Ashwagandha two times per day. After eight weeks, they showed significant improvement in short- and long-term memory, were able to process information better, and were more efficient in completing tasks.[7]

PREPARATION, SOURCING, AND DOSAGE

The most common way to purchase Ashwagandha is in a powder, capsules, tincture, or as pieces of dried root. If using the dried root, we recommend making your own decoction. To do this, simply add one teaspoon of root per eight ounces or one cup of water into a slow cooker or crockpot. Let steep for a few hours, strain, and drink. If using the powder, start with one to two teaspoons per day or about 200 to 500 milligrams. Always check in with your body periodically before jumping to a higher dosage too soon. You can slowly build up to approximately 1.2 grams per day if needed.

While the root can be taken on its own, we strongly recommend combining it with other herbs to create a formula unique to your body's needs. Due to the bitter nature of the root, try combining it with either cooling foods or herbs (plant-based milk, ghee, etc.). Some find it hard to digest on its own. If you find yourself feeling a bit nauseous after taking it, mix it with food or add it into a nourishing beverage. We love mixing it with carminatives (warming, digestive supportive herbs) like nutmeg, cardamom, or cinnamon to avoid a tummy ache. As a gentle and nourishing Adaptogen, Ashwagandha is safe in both short and long-term use. Look for Ashwagandha sourced from India, its country of origin, and always go for organic to avoid pesticides.

REAL-LIFE WAYS TO BENEFIT FROM ASHWAGANDHA

- *For stress:* Make a traditional decoction with milk, ghee, and honey and take before bed to unwind and prepare for sleep. For a similar plant-based alternative, use your nut milk of choice, coconut oil, and a dash of maple syrup.

- *For longevity:* Mix the root powder with carminative herbs such as cinnamon and cardamom for a longevity tonic day or night.

- *For brain:* Scoop powder into a smoothie or tea to help turn on your brain in the morning or afternoon.

Restore *(Stress and Mood)* Case Study

A woman struggling with autoimmune disease, thyroiditis, inflammatory polyarthritis, and ovarian cysts shared her healing story with us. After being hospitalized four times in one year, she felt debilitated and pushed to her body's limit. She added Ashwagandha to her morning coffee for a few months and then took a few weeks off. After a month without the Ashwagandha, her hormones "went out of whack." Estrogen levels skyrocketed, and she developed ovarian cysts and torsions which led to crippling pain in her abdomen that radiated throughout her body. Her joints were on fire. Realizing the Ashwagandha in her coffee was the one piece of her life that had shifted, she swiftly added the Ashwagandha back into her morning routine. Within a few weeks, her joint pain was significantly reduced. After a few months, she had complete pain relief again. She continues to drink her Adaptogenic coffee every morning and has energy throughout the day while living pain-free.

REISHI

Full legal name: *Ganoderma lucidum* from the *Ganoderma* family

Nicknames: Queen of mushrooms, lingzhi, the mushroom/elixir of immortality, the ten-thousand-year mushroom, and varnished conk mushroom

Power hub: Mushroom fruiting body

Home: Worldwide

Energetics: Warm, neutral to slightly dry

Helpful with:

1. Stress
2. Longevity
3. Immunity

Comes with:

- Four hundred biologically active constituents, including:
  - Polysaccharides 1,3, 1,6 beta-d-glucans
  - Triterpenes: ganodermanontriol, Ganoderic acid
  - Lingzhi-9 protein

Common uses: Before bed, or when feeling tired for any reason (illness or stress)

Best friends: Cacao, Cordyceps, Ashwagandha, Tulsi, cinnamon, rose hips, and other foods high in Vitamin C

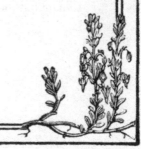

A BRIEF HISTORY: The #1 Rated "Herb" that Is Actually a Mushroom

Reishi is the most sacred of all Adaptogens. It was once reserved only for emperors and gods and known as the elixir of immortality. In the emperor's palace in ancient China, it's sculpted in archways and placed in doorways as a symbol of good luck and good health. It's been a treasured talisman and potent medicine in China for over four thousand years. One of its many names is the ten-thousand-year mushroom, which refers to the belief that it will help you live for 10,000 years. Its shiny, shelf-like appearance (looks like it has a resin or polish on it, totally naturally) is rare in nature. Legends say that if commoners in China found Reishi in the wild, it was forbidden to keep it for themselves. Chinese law mandated that any foraged Reishi must be delivered to the palace for use by royalty.

In TCM, there are 365 ingredients of the *Herbal Classic* Materia Medica. All herbs are divided into three grades: superior, average, and fair. Superior herbs are the most medicinally potent while having no negative side effects. Of all herbs in the *Classic*, Reishi is given first place (even above Ginseng).

Note that when reading ancient texts and materia medicas, Reishi has been conflated with many similar species in the Ganoderma family, including *Ganoderma tsugae*, *Ganoderma sinense*, and *Ganoderma lingzhi*.

Taxonomy and Naming of Species

Mushroom and fungi taxonomy is an ongoing and never-ending process. Today, mushroom DNA barcoding is used as an identification method. Yet before that process was discovered and used, many mushrooms were lumped into the same category if they looked similar or showed similar benefits in humans. Reishi is a prime example of this happening. Several clinical papers written before DNA barcoding discussed the use of *Ganoderma lucidum* when they were actually using *tsugae* or *lingzhi*.

Research, identification, and discovery is constantly improving and evolving. During our lifetime alone, Cordyceps alone has changed its name three times! As poor identification and cultivation improve, it's highly likely that the number of different varieties of each Adaptogen will continue to evolve and improve within the same genus. An example of this is with mushroom identification. One of the many ways to identify mushrooms is to take spore prints of the same species to find a strain that grows the most efficiently. As you are cloning, you can continue to use the stronger and better spores and cultivate those. Even with a standard Oyster mushroom, there can be hundreds of different oyster mushroom varieties from them.

HELPFUL WITH STRESS

Reishi is best known for its gentle ability to unwind the nervous system. It helps prepare you for a deep night of rest due to its normalizing and balancing effect of helping your body adapt to stress and maintain a state of equilibrium. Yet how it helps alleviate symptoms of stress is unique from other nervines. Reishi will never knock you out. In fact, it's fine to take Reishi any time of day to gently relieve stress and calm your system. The anxiety relief from Reishi is a short-term action, which builds energy in the long term. Just like a good night of rest gives you more energy the next day, Reishi allows your system to destress, bringing greater vitality in the long run.

One study looked at Reishi's effect on chronic fatigue syndrome, a state where the body has been pushed beyond acute stress. In this clinical trial, the treatment group was given two grams of an aqueous (water) extract of Reishi per day, divided into four, half-gram doses, versus a placebo. Results showed that those taking Reishi had a significant reduction in fatigue markers and experienced an improvement in quality of life, with minimal-to-no side effects.[8]

HELPFUL FOR LONGEVITY

Reishi appeared in writings as early as the 16th century. One of the early examples is in the Pen Ts'ao Kang Mu pharmacopeia, where Li Shih-chen wrote, "[Reishi] positively affects the life-energy, or Qi of the heart, repairing the chest area and benefiting those who have a knotted and tight chest. Taken over a long period of time, the agility of your body will not cease, and the years are lengthened to those of the Immortal Fairies." Immortal Fairies or not, Reishi is shown to support many parts of your body responsible for longevity. It has long been associated with the heart, as a cardiovascular tonic. The traditional stories of Reishi for chest and heart concerns have been further backed by modern research.[9]

Reishi has been well studied for its hepatoprotective qualities, its ability to protect the liver. Picture the filter of a sink. If it is clogged, the rest of the sink will fill up with dirty water and cause a whole mess. Similarly, if our internal filter is clogged, our body is weighed down. A host of symptoms may arise from the liver performing suboptimally.

One gold-standard study looked at how Reishi triterpenes and polysaccharides affect liver health. For six months, one group was given Reishi extract and the other a placebo. Most notably, Reishi reversed the participants' mild fatty liver condition back to a normal state, and those who took Reishi had substantially more antioxidants and beneficial liver enzymes, confirming Reishi's powerful liver-protective benefits via activating antioxidants and reducing oxidative stress.[10]

HELPFUL WITH IMMUNITY

Reishi is anti-inflammatory, anti-allergic, antiviral, antibacterial, antifungal, and even anti-cancer—all great things for immunity. Regulating inflammation is foundational to a healthy body. On the flip side, chronic inflammation is at the root of many common diseases. Reishi's anti-inflammatory properties can target inflammatory cytokines and modulate the immune system based on your body's needs.[11] This classic Adaptogenic regulation of the immune system makes Reishi a supremely effective option for a range of immunocompromised conditions.

Radiation, much like excess sunlight, damages DNA and kills cells, including white blood cells. White blood cells are the part of our immune system responsible for protecting the body against infectious diseases and foreign invaders, and a lack of them weakens our immune system, making us more vulnerable and susceptible to disease. Multiple studies show that Reishi prevents our number of white blood cells from decreasing.[12] This is particularly helpful for people going through radiation therapy but is essentially relevant for anyone interested in protecting against daily DNA damage.

There have been many cases of "spontaneous" remission in cancer patients using Reishi extracts.[13] We believe it is fully due to Reishi's "superpowers" of having more identified immunomodulating polysaccharides and triterpenes than any other mushroom and an ability to modulate the immune system. It is among the safest of all Adaptogens to take daily for long-term immune support.

On top of this support for a balanced, strong, and vital immune system, Reishi also helps with seasonal allergies through regulation of Th1/Th2. By essentially making our antibodies more effective and efficient, Reishi offers antihistamine benefits and can help prevent allergies from coming on in the first place.[14]

PREPARATION, SOURCING, AND DOSAGE

Like all functional mushrooms, the gold standard is to use log-grown, fruiting bodies that have been properly extracted. Extracts should be aqueous (decoction), alcohol (tincture), or both (dual extract). Unfortunately, according to a study published in the credible *Nature* publication, 74 percent of Reishi products in the U.S. didn't contain authentic Reishi.[15] It is so important to find trusted brands that offer real ingredients. The mushroom marketplace is getting more crowded by the day, so vetting brands and understanding how to properly read labels is key.

We recommend starting with 500 milligrams per day of a dual-extracted, log-grown Reishi fruiting body. The highest dose we recommend is 4 grams per day; some research has been done with six grams per day but that is not necessary for most. The amount needed will depend on your body's needs—both physical factors like gut and liver health, as well as things like how stressed you are. Start small and build up by about 500 milligrams every five to seven days until you find the dose that feels right for you. Remember that more is not always better!

Beyond dosage, ensure you are getting USDA-certified organic mushrooms. Fungi are bio accumulators and can absorb a lot from the environment or substrate they are grown in. To further ensure a high-quality product, aim to find mushrooms that have been third-party tested for things like mycotoxins, irradiation, and heavy metals.

REAL-LIFE WAYS TO BENEFIT FROM REISHI

- *For stress:* Drink Reishi decoction in the evening instead of a glass of red wine to calm your nervous system and prepare your body for a deep night of rest.

- *For longevity:* Add extracted Reishi powder to tea or coffee to bring more balance and calm into the day. If older, sip daily to support energy and the immune system.

- *For immunity:* Add slices of dried Reishi root into a stew or broth, let simmer overnight, and eat or drink before, during, or after an illness.

TULSI

Full legal name: *Ocimum sanctum* from the *Lamiaceae* (mint) family

Nicknames: Holy basil, matchless one, incomparable one

Power hub: Leaf (occasionally lends its flowers or root)

Home: Primarily India but found across Asia and in Central and South America

Energetics: Warming and cooling, slightly dry

Helpful with:

1. Stress
2. Longevity
3. Mood

Comes with:

- Rosmarinic acid
- Eugenol
- Oleanolic acid
- Ursolic acid
- Apigenin
- Carnosic acid
- Flavonoids: orientin and vicenin
- β-caryophyllene
- Carotenoids

Common uses: Chilling, meditating, yin yoga, and breathwork

Best friends: Reishi, Ashwagandha, black pepper, ginger, and hawthorn berry

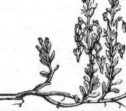

A BRIEF HISTORY: A Leaf to
Worship, Wear, and Heal

The holiest of Adaptogens, Tulsi is the most sacred plant in Hinduism. It's thought to increase prana or life force and has revered names including "goddess incarnated in plant form." Part of its holiness comes from it being tridoshic, which means that it's beneficial for all *doshas*, or body types, in Ayurvedic medicine. It was traditionally grown in temple courtyards as an homage to Lakshmi, the goddess of wealth, and Vishnu, the god of absolute consciousness.

Used and revered for over five thousand years in Ayurveda, it's considered one of India's most powerful herbs. In fact, a Hindu family's home is considered incomplete without a Tulsi plant. They place it on the altar, give it a specially built structure with images of deities on all sides, or grow it in the gardens of their home. Praying to Tulsi is a way of worshipping the gods—the divine alive within the leaves—and it is usually prayed over twice a day, in the morning and evening. A garland made of Tulsi is a valuable spiritual offering.

With this plant's deep history come many myths and legends. One claims the plant is an incarnation of a princess. Another tells that Lord Krishna was weighed in gold, and the only thing that could tip the scales of worth was a single Tulsi leaf.

Apart from its deeply religious significance, Tulsi has been used as a prized medicinal plant. It's called "the elixir of life" and "bridge between Heaven and Earth," much like Reishi in TCM. It's used to treat everything from the common cold and digestive complaints to heart disease, malaria, and forms of poisoning. Modern research shows it's effective against diabetes, hypertension, cancers, and bronchitis.[16] A plant of mind, body, and spirit, Tulsi is versatile in its healing potential physically and spiritually.

There are over 100 varieties of Tulsi, but two are the most used and available: Rama Tulsi (green leaf) or Krishna Tulsi (purple leaf). Both varieties now have modern research to confirm their many beneficial compounds for whole-body health.[17]

HELPFUL WITH STRESS

As a nervine, Tulsi primarily helps your body adapt to stressors and new demands. Physically, it protects the heart from stress, particularly when anxiety leads to high blood pressure. Mentally, it helps balance mood, lifts mental fog, and promotes memory. And spiritually, it soothes depression, promotes joy, and harmonizes the chakras.

In a 2016 study, rats given Tulsi for 16 consecutive days showed that Tulsi was able to inhibit or stop cortisol release, confirming its effectiveness in the management of stress.[18]

Another trial in which people with generalized anxiety disorder (GAD) were given 500 milligram capsules of Tulsi two times per day found that Tulsi significantly attenuated GAD and correlated stress and depression, the results logged in a standard questionnaire given to assess psychological state. It also improved people's willingness to try new treatments, making it a promising anxiolytic treatment for GAD.[19]

HELPFUL FOR LONGEVITY

One of Tulsi's key compounds is the essential oil eugenol. Much of the longevity research focuses on this compound, and Indian scientists have found it positively affects the immune, reproductive, cardiovascular, urinary, gastric, and central nervous systems.[20] Other essential oils of Tulsi (including carvacrol, usolic acid, β-caryophyllene, and rosmarinic acid) are also anti-inflammatory. Together these oils protect the digestive system and protect against stress.[21]

In a double-blind, randomized, controlled trial, volunteers who took 300 milligram capsules of Tulsi extract for four weeks showed a statistically significant change in levels of immune factors such as Th1 and Th2 cytokines, T-helper and T-cytotoxic cells, B-cells, and NK-cells compared to the placebo group. Tulsi was found to be immunomodulatory, able to stimulate or down-regulate immune cells based on the needs of the individual. This profound balancing effect on the immune system makes it a potent longevity herb.[22]

Preliminary research suggests Tulsi could potentially help prevent and treat cancer. Phytochemicals in Tulsi leaves including eugenol and rosmarinic acid have been shown to prevent radiation-induced DNA damage, and Tulsi leaves have chemoprotective and radioprotective properties which have shown to be highly beneficial against cancer.[23] With free-radical scavenging and anti-inflammatory abilities, Tulsi leaves are protective against the major diseases of the body, further confirming its place as a superior ally for longevity.[24]

HELPFUL WITH MOOD

While we often associate mood with brain or mental health, mood is regulated systemically through your body. New research confirms the gut or microbiome is the body's second brain, primarily because of the sheer number of neurons located in the gut lining. While the gut doesn't have brain waves, it does have about 100 million nerve cells of the same kind found in the brain.

Mental illness is of increasing concern in today's world. The use of pharmaceuticals to treat depression and anxiety is vast and growing by the day. A study comparing Tulsi to a common class of pharmaceutical antidepressants called Imipramine showed that Tulsi at a dose of 500 milligrams per kilogram of body weight had comparable antidepressant activity to Imipramine, without the laundry list of side effects.[25] Tulsi further comes with a host of other benefits to mood, longevity, stress, anxiety, and depression.[26]

Mints are famous for being beneficial to digestion and gut health, and Tulsi, which is in the Lamiaceae or mint family, is no exception. Like peppermint or spearmint, the essential oils in Tulsi relieve acute symptoms of stomach upset, reduce the length and severity of abdominal pain, and act as antispasmodics to ease cramping or general stomach upset.

Beyond the mint family benefits, Tulsi has shown to be effective in treating H. pylori and associated stomach ulcers. This is profound because H. pylori is a bacteria present in almost 50 percent of all people on the planet. H. pylori can damage stomach tissue, cause inflammation, gastritis, and in bad cases, lead to stomach cancer. In a four-week trial, patients with ulcers who were given antibiotics (standard treatment) with Tulsi and coconut oil had 100 percent eradication of H. pylori compared to 50 percent eradication in the placebo. Plus, other symptoms from the ulcers such as pain were reduced in those taking Tulsi.[27]

From the gut to the brain, Tulsi supports both centers of neuronal activity and thus, mood. It's a powerful ally to lift the mood from the root of the potential problem. More than being a bandage, it helps to relieve the body of inflammation, pain, and depressive thoughts, and heal the gut and the mind to bring about a greater sense of mental ease and joy.

PREPARATION, SOURCING, AND DOSAGE

You can find Tulsi in many forms, most commonly as capsules, tincture, powder, or whole dried leaf. Since it is an Ayurvedic herb, the highest quality products should come from India. An effective starting dose in a capsule or dried powder is 300 to 500 milligrams per day of extracted leaves. If using a tincture, we recommend starting with 40 to 60 drops (about one to two dropperfuls) up to three times per day. The dried herb is a great way to get to know the plant and gives you much flexibility in terms of use. The simplest way to use whole or dried Tulsi leaves is by making an infusion. Boil water and pour one cup (or eight ounces) over one tablespoon of herb. Let it steep for 20 to 30 minutes, or as long as overnight for a stronger medicinal tea. Fresh Tulsi leaves can also be used in cooking to flavor meals, much like classic culinary basil. To keep the medicinal compounds in cooking, avoid frying the leaves. Instead, try steaming or boiling.

REAL-LIFE WAYS TO BENEFIT FROM TULSI

- *For stress:* Drink a daily infusion of leaves to calm the nervous system.

- *For longevity:* Add powder into smoothies for daily support.

- *For gut health:* Steep a tea of Tulsi leaves to soothe digestive upset.

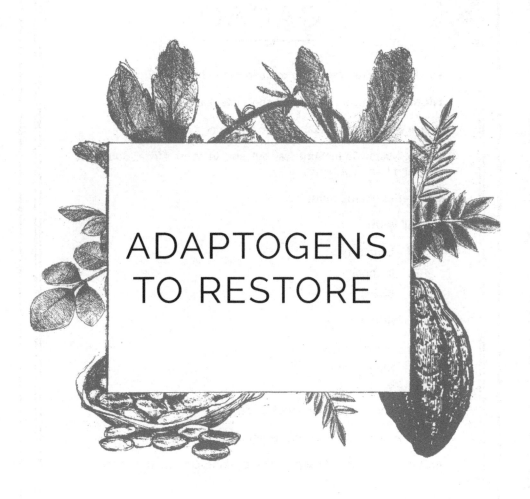

ADAPTOGENS TO RESTORE

FOR LONGEVITY AND WELL-BEING

CACAO

Full legal name: *Theobroma cacao* from the house of fruit trees

Nicknames: Cocoa, coco bean, chocolate, kakaw, xocolatl

Power hub: Edible nut, also called a bean or a seed

Home: Mainly South America, but also in West Africa, Southeast Asia, and Central America

Energetics: Warm, moist

Helpful with:

1. Longevity
2. Immunity
3. Brain

Comes with:

- Theobromine
- Magnesium
- Tryptophan
- Phenylethylamine (PEA)

Common uses: Evenings and ceremonial occasions

Best friends: Reishi, Mucuna, vanilla, cayenne, cinnamon, and coconut

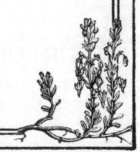

A BRIEF HISTORY: From Currency to the World's Most Popular Nut

Cacao has been used as a currency, mood enhancer, love drug, sign of prosperity, and is the world's most complex food. It is the oldest Adaptogen with a recorded history of human use. People have been trading, drinking, and praying over this bean for 15,000 years! Cacao is derived from *kakaw* in ancient Zoque, the language of the Olmec people of Mesoamerica, the first Cacao-loving civilization. The Olmecs passed the tradition of Cacao use to the Mayans, who shared it with the Aztecs, who revered the bean so highly that they began using it for trade, where it remained a valid currency in Mexico until 1887. Beyond the Cacao trade, the bean was fermented, dried, roasted, ground into a paste, and mixed with water and spices to create a powerful tonic. Cacao was used in ceremonies for its heart-opening and euphoria exhibiting properties. Many experienced a "high" from drinking it, putting it into a class of sacred plants. Its magical effects make it both a religious and status symbol.

It took several hundred years, ocean crossings, and a chemist to turn Cacao into a chocolate bar. In August 1502, Christopher Columbus robbed a Mayan trading ship and stole their Cacao. He had seen the local praise of the beans, so even though he was unaware of their benefits, he stole enough to bring back to Europe. After years of Cacao circulating across Europe, two chemists in the 1800s helped make it into chocolate bars. First, the Dutch Coenraad Johannes van Houten invented the "Dutch process" to press the fats from the bean, making the full Cacao into the more processed cocoa powder sold in stores. Then the Swiss chemist Henri Nestlé—founder of Nestlé—tinkered with the bean, combining it with milk and sugar. And just like that, modern-day chocolate was born! The word "chocolate" comes from the Aztec word "xocoatl," meaning "bitter water." Even though the bitterness is taken away by the milk and sugars, the name remains.

As the world's most popular nut, Cacao, is still revered today for the relaxation, energy, joy, and love that was felt from indulging in it thousands of years ago. Cacao's traditional value is now confirmed by scientific research. It contains 1,200 active compounds that support your brain, heart, immune system, and well-being in a multitude of ways.[1]

HELPFUL FOR LONGEVITY

With its heart-supporting minerals and antioxidants, Cacao has long been associated with longevity. A 2005 study from University Hospital in Zurich found that just a few squares (about three ounces) of at least 74 percent dark chocolate daily may significantly reduce the risk of serious heart disease and that consuming about 1.5 ounces of it increased arterial blood flow for eight hours. The results don't stand with normal milk or white chocolate that's full of sugar. No wonder the Swiss live so long and eat so much chocolate!

Cacao also contains more magnesium than any other natural food source. This important mineral is involved in over 300 critical functions in your body, including helping to regulate blood sugar and allowing us to relax on a cellular level.[2] Yet despite being one of the most essential minerals in the human body, about 75 percent of the U.S. population is deficient in it. A healthy heart is key to longevity, and heart muscles rely on magnesium to function optimally. Magnesium reduces hypertension and arrhythmia, dilates blood vessels to stop heart spasming, breaks up blood clots, and controls the action of calcium to keep a proper balance of contraction and relaxation of the cells. In knowing the relationship between heart health and magnesium, it makes sense that Cacao is a symbol of love.

HELPFUL FOR IMMUNITY

Ten percent of Cacao's weight is antioxidants. This means it contains more antioxidants than blueberries, Goji, red wine, and pomegranates combined! Cacao's antioxidants known as polyphenols and flavanols are present from its black color pigments.[3] They are anti-inflammatory, nerve protective, and skin protective, and are supportive of cognition and mood.[4] Another antioxidant found in Cacao is Vitamin C, which has been found to prevent and treat infections. Vitamin C is also one of the first recommended supplements when you're under the weather.

In an in vivo study done in 2016 in Japan, two groups of people were given an injection of a strain of the human influenza (flu) virus. One group was given Cacao powder three weeks before and three weeks after the injection, the other group a placebo. The group taking Cacao showed increased natural killer cell activity and stronger protection against the virus.[5]

HELPFUL FOR THE BRAIN

A cognitive powerhouse, Cacao contains phytonutrients that protect and enhance the brain, including caffeine's less aggressive "sister nutrient," theobromine. Fun fact: "Theobroma" is Greek for "food of the gods." Caffeine and theobromine are both alkaloids, so they are similar in chemical structure, but there are some major differences in the way they affect our bodies. Theobromine is less stimulating than caffeine and has a longer-lasting, gentler effect on your body. Caffeine stimulates the nervous system (jitters, anyone?), while theobromine stimulates the cardiovascular system and blood flow. More blood flow to the brain means more energy to think and perform. A 2016 study from Kanazawa University in Japan proved that theobromine increased motor learning in mice.[6] Another 2019 study from the University of Milan in Italy showed that theobromine has a neuroprotective action on the brain. In brief, theobromine is what coffee wishes it was![7]

Beyond theobromine, Cacao contains two important neurotransmitters for the brain. The first, anandamide (N-arachidonoyl ethanolamide), is a cannabinoid (yes, the same group of compounds found in cannabis!). It's known to lighten the mood, help lift depressive thoughts, and stimulate parts of the brain associated with motivation.[8] The second neurotransmitter, phenylethylamine (PEA), activates parts of our brain associated with concentration, perception, and pleasure. PEA is increased when we're in love and depleted when we're depressed. It's also the compound behind the infamous "Cacao flow," where time seems to slip away and you get "in the zone." PEA is destroyed by heat, which happens in the process of turning Cacao into cocoa, so always look for *Cacao* over *cocoa* to get those pleasure benefits.

PREPARATION, SOURCING, AND DOSAGE

Sourcing and quality are key when it comes to Cacao. Always look for *Cacao* over *cocoa*. High-quality Cacao will be less unprocessed and richer with its 1,200 phytonutrients. Always look for organic Cacao because of the many beneficial minerals (magnesium!) come from the soil it's grown in. If the soil is depleted or full of pesticides and heavy metals, your Cacao will be, too. If you're using pure Cacao beans, they should be waxy and oily. If they're moldy, rubbery, or smoky smelling or tasting, they've gone bad.

For health and humanitarian reasons, avoid Cacao from West Africa, where it is often grown in monocultures, which are bad for the soil and nutrient density. This region also is often accused of using child labor. Instead, the highest quality Cacao usually comes from Ecuador or Peru, with the next-best region being the Caribbean. As long as you're getting properly sourced, minimally processed, organic Cacao, you're set!

As for dosage, Cacao is more of a food, so eat or nibble on it as your body craves and desires. Ceremonial doses start around 10 grams and go up to around 40 to 50 grams for those who have a longer history and experience with the plant. We find that 15 to 20 mg is a powerful and potent dose if used consistently for its functional benefits.

REAL-LIFE WAYS TO BENEFIT FROM CACAO

- *For longevity:* Drink as a coffee or energy drink substitute to limit daily caffeine consumption and improve whole-body wellness.

- *For brain:* Turn into raw chocolate and add other brain-boosting buddies like Mucuna, Lion's Mane, and Rhodiola for a mood enhancer (and love potion).

- *For stress:* Drink as an evening ritual instead of red wine to let the nervous system know it's time to unwind and rest. Best paired with Reishi and Ashwagandha for this purpose.

Restore *(Stress and Mood)* Case Study

There are three famous stories about the oldest women who have ever lived. The oldest, a 127-year-old from Mexico, the second a 122.5-year-old French woman, and lastly a 121-year-old Italian woman. All three of them, upon being asked their secret to longevity, had the same answer: Cacao. The Mexican woman's grandchildren called her a true fighter. She was active her entire life, even said to be weaving until the last two years of life. The French woman smoked cigarettes her entire life, offsetting it with about two pounds of chocolate each week. She rarely took medications but loved rituals. She was cycling until age 100, had a steady skincare regimen focused on olive oil, and would start each morning with prayer. The Italian woman was known for her positive attitude and eating chocolate every day. The power of Cacao and its longevity benefits are seen through each of these women's miraculously long, happy, and healthy lives.

GYNOSTEMMA

Full legal name: *Gynostemma pentaphyllum* from the *Cucurbitaceae* (cucumber) family

Nicknames: Miracle grass/tea/herb, sweet tea vine, southern or poor man's Ginseng (although not a real Ginseng)

Power hub: Leaf

Home: Mountains of China, occasionally found in Japan, Korea, and Vietnam

Energetics: Neutral, neutral

Helpful with:

1. Longevity
2. Endurance
3. Stress

Comes with:

- Triterpenoid saponins: gypenosides
- Polysaccharides (PGPs, GPTP-3)[9]
- Antioxidants: SOD (superoxide dismutase)
- Actiponin
- Glutathione

Common uses: Mornings and afternoons at work

Best friends: Gotu Kola, Goji, jasmine, green tea, and peppermint

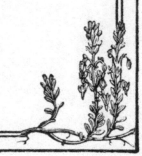

A BRIEF HISTORY: The Mountains
Vine for Centenarians

As the legend goes, a servant of the Chinese emperor Fu Shou was boiling water outside one day. The leaves of a nearby vine fell into the water and began to steep. Unknowingly, this created the first infusion of the Gynostemma leaf. The emperor drank the infused water with much enjoyment. He commented that it was a delightful mix of refreshing, bitter, and sweet. Little did he know at the time that this experience would pave the way to the discovery of the "miracle herb." From its humble start, Gynostemma went on to become a revered medicine for its longevity, endurance, and stress benefits. Rumors spread that those who drank the tea would live a long and healthy life.

Native to altitudes of up to 10,000 feet in China, Gynostemma is a relative to common fruits like cucumber and melons. But unlike these fruits, it does not bear edible fruit, and instead, the leaves hold the medicine. Locals have been using the five-leafed plant for hundreds of years, both eaten raw and steeped as tea. Its slightly sweet taste gave it a place as a sugar substitute with a low-glycemic profile.

Gynostemma can be thought of as a cure-all. It's anti-aging, anti-inflammatory, antioxidant, and anti-cancer. It also has a calming effect on the heart and mind. Some use it for its digestive and respiratory system support, while others take it for liver health, cholesterol levels, bone health, and their immune system.

In the 1960s, the herb gained popularity in the West after the discovery of a special group of compounds in the leaf. These triterpenoid saponins are nearly identical to those found in the revered Asian Ginseng. As such, both plants help improve resistance to stress, support cholesterol buildup, and fight free radicals. The difference is that Gynostemma has a gentle and calming effect on the nervous system, whereas Ginseng is quite stimulating. Gynostemma is also easier to find and cheaper, so it is sometimes called "poor man's Ginseng." Its value was further confirmed through a nationwide census in China of the 1970s that identified a mountainous community in the Guizhou province with the largest percentage of people living over 100 years old. Their secret? Gynostemma.

HELPFUL WITH LONGEVITY

Gynostemma's most potent medicinal effects come from saponins and antioxidants. Over 230 compounds have been isolated from Gynostemma, 189 of which are saponins.[10] This makes it the highest saponin-containing plant in the world, over four times that found in Ginseng. The particular kind of saponins present are called gypenosides, which are similar to the ginsenosides found in Ginseng (and some even convert to ginsenosides in your body). They're immunomodulating (able to stimulate or suppress immune activity as needed), anti-inflammatory, and antioxidant.[11] Astoundingly, studies on Gynostemma in conjunction with radiotherapy in cancer have found that Gynostemma may be used as a radioprotector, meaning it protects tissues of the body from the toxic side effects of radiation.[12] This offers huge potential for cancer patients who undergo radiation therapy by possibly saving them from the negative side effects of that treatment.[13]

Gynostemma's other compounds include sterols, antioxidants, and polysaccharides. The compounds responsible for Gynostemma's anti-aging reputation are the antioxidants SOD and glutathione. They work together with the saponins to prevent oxidative damage and support balance, memory, and fatigue.

Another important component to a long, healthy life is ensuring our body can utilize its energy input. We're talking about sugar. Blood sugar balance is critical to our body's ability to have the right fuel it needs, at the proper dose and time, to function optimally. In combination with exercise and good diet, Gynostemma has been shown to regulate insulin production and help stabilize blood sugar levels.[14] This is beneficial for those with type 2 diabetes and those who struggle with weight imbalance.

Whether over- or underweight, this herb can help bring your body back to its normal weight. Many common heart diseases originate from an imbalance in blood sugar metabolism, and proper insulin balance is a key preventative measure for heart disease. A healthy blood-sugar balance, leading to heart health, sets a strong foundation for longevity.

HELPFUL FOR ENDURANCE

Gynostemma contains unique compounds known as Polysaccharides from *Gynostemma pentaphyllum* (PGPs). Among its benefits is anti-fatigue. An animal study conducted to test the physical stamina benefits of Gynostemma found that after 30 days of taking Gynostemma, rats in a forced swim test showed that PGP had three levels of anti-fatigue benefits. First, it directly extended the exhaustive swimming time of the rats. Second, it decreased blood lactic acid (BLA) and blood urea nitrogen (BUN), which is important, because if there is too much BLA and BUN in the system, it can lead to fatigue. Lastly, PGP increased their hemoglobin, liver glycogen, and muscle glycogen concentrations. Glycogen is a sugar and a form of fuel that your body uses when exercising. The more glycogen available for use, the longer your body can exercise without burning out.[15] It's no wonder this leaf has been a popular endurance aid for athletes. The combination of building lean muscle while reducing fatigue makes it an athlete's dream.

HELPFUL WITH STRESS

The body is a constantly calibrating machine, where there is a small threshold of several factors that it must stay within for optimal function—temperature, blood pressure, heart rate, and the list goes on. When a stressor occurs, it instantly throws your body out of this range, and essentially, out of whack. Your body is then on a mission to return to a state of homeostasis as quickly as possible, because when pushed beyond its balanced state, disease, inflammation, and illness set in. Thus, when we talk about stress, balance and homeostasis are integral.

Gynostemma has the unique ability to activate the enzyme AMP-activated protein kinase (AMPK). AMPK is a major cellular regulator that helps the body balance energy input and output. Specifically, it regulates your body's levels of lipids (fats), glucose (sugar), and biological energy homeostasis.[16] The need for balance and homeostasis is critical in cases of stress to ensure your body recovers quickly and doesn't stay in an extended state of stress. Many studies have been done on the relationship of AMPK in stress.[17,18,19] One placebo-controlled, double-blind study found that the group of individuals with chronic stress and anxiety who were exposed to repetitive stress had lower anxiety and reduced psychological stress compared to the placebo group.[20]

PREPARATION, SOURCING, AND DOSAGE

Gynostemma is most commonly sold in the form of dried leaves, capsules, tinctures, and powders. Regardless of the form used, the most important thing to look for is quality. Always purchase organic Gynostemma that has ideally been third-party lab tested to ensure the product is devoid of common contaminants like heavy metals and pesticides.

Gynostemma is one of the few Adaptogens that can easily be grown at home. If growing your own, we encourage also trying to make your own extraction. Simply make an infusion using one to two tablespoons of dried leaves to one cup of hot water, and steep for approximately 15 minutes. Strain out the leaves and drink up to three cups per day. (Pro tip: the tea is ready when it turns a green/brown color and resembles the taste of green tea.)

If using a tincture, an effective starting dose is 80 to 120 drops (about two to three dropperfuls) up to three times per day. If using an extract, take 10 to 150 milligrams per day, divided into two or three doses. If using the dried leaf as a powder, there is a wide range of dosing, anywhere from 1 to 10 grams per day. Our recommendation is to start small, with one to two grams per day, and slowly build up after about a week. The next week, increase the dose to three to four grams per day, divided into two doses. For best results, take 30 minutes apart from meals, which is a good rule of thumb with all liquid Adaptogens.

Since Gynostemma leaf is edible, you can also experiment with eating the leaf in recipes. Try making it into a pesto, sauteing with other vegetables, or adding it into a mixed green salad.

REAL-LIFE WAYS TO BENEFIT FROM GYNOSTEMMA

- *For longevity:* Make a tea with the dried leaves to replace a morning or midafternoon cup of green tea.

- *For endurance:* Add fresh leaves to a medicinal pesto—put on your favorite post-workout meal for an herbal enhanced, tonifying, and nourishing recovery meal to support long-term endurance.

- *For stress:* Add powder to tea (our favorite is with peppermint) or a smoothie to add calm energy to your day.

MORINGA

Full legal name: *Moringa oleifera* from the *Moringaceae* family

Nicknames: Tree of life, and horseradish/drumstick/benzolive/miracle/wonder tree

Power hub: Leaf (occasionally the root and seed pods are used)

Home: Tropical and subtropical climates, including Africa, Southeast Asia, and the tropical Americas

Energetics: Neutral, neutral

Helpful with:

1. Longevity
2. Mood
3. Beauty

Comes with:

- Antioxidant properties:
  - Polyphenolic flavonoids: quercetin, glucosinolates, and kaempferol glycosides
- Zeatin, caffeoylquinic acid, beta-sitosterol
- Carotenoids: Beta-carotene
- Essential amino acids
- Minerals: iron, potassium, calcium, manganese, boron, chromium
- Vitamins A, B, C, and E

Common uses: When you're starting to get hangry

Best friends: Oat straw, nettle, spearmint, sage, ghee, or other healthy fats

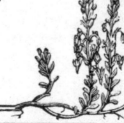

A BRIEF HISTORY: A Medicine Cabinet In a Tree

Moringa is referred to as the "miracle tree" or "tree of life." It has an incredible nutrient profile and a wide range of uses that live up to its lofty nicknames. While it's most commonly used for its Adaptogenic leaves, almost every part of the tree is used for food or medicine. Traditionally, the bark, flowers, seeds, pods, and roots were utilized. The roots get made into a horseradish flavored condiment. The seeds are pressed to make a medicinal oil. The flowers are made into honey to support respiratory ailments. The root is powdered and used as a mineral-rich supplement. Unripened pods are cooked in curries to prevent intestinal worms. The bark is used as a cure for eye and ear infections. In particular, the leaves, the Adaptogenic part of the tree, have a wide range of uses themselves. They can be eaten raw, made into tea, or applied topically to heal skin ailments. They are even used as a water purifier because of their antibacterial properties.

Moringa's use dates back 5,000 years in Ayurveda and Unani (ancient Greek) systems of medicine, and for hundreds of years in Africa to help fight malnutrition. In Ethiopia, the Konso people rely on Moringa leaves as a staple food source. In India, the pods are consumed and packaged as a trade item. In West Africa, the leaves are used to make sauces. Of the 13 species in the Moringa family, the *oleifera* is the easiest to propagate, reproduce, and grow, making it a choice tree to proliferate in areas where food security is of peak concern.

Moringa is packed with an astonishing amount of nutrients. It has minerals like iron and potassium, an impressive range of antioxidants, amino acids, vitamin C, and various phenolics, making it beneficial for sleep, heart health, kidneys, liver, blood, the pancreas, and more. Its many pharmacological actions include pain-relieving, anti-inflammatory, anti-asthmatic, antiulcer, and antispasmodic, antibacterial, antihyperglycemic, antioxidant, and anti-cancer. The cherry on top is its safety profile. Since it is a food-like herb, it has been found to be extremely safe in nearly all bodies and conditions.[21] All in all, Moringa is easy to grow, widely available, affordable, and has promising efficacy with minimal side effects.

HELPFUL WITH LONGEVITY

Ensuring that all cells, tissues, and organs have enough nutrients is critical for longevity. With deficiencies, cells begin to die, and organs slow down or can't function optimally. This leads to exhaustion, headaches, digestive issues, and vulnerability to sickness, making nutrition and longevity go hand in hand. After all, everything we feed our body becomes the nutrient building blocks for all systems to function, and Moringa happens to be one of the most nutrient-dense foods in the world.

Moringa leaves have double the amount of protein per 100 grams as yogurt (8.3 grams to yogurt's 3.8 grams). It has four times the calcium as milk (434 milligrams to whole cow milk's 120 milligrams), and approximately the same amount of potassium as a banana (404 mg to banana's 376 milligrams). It even has about the same amount of vitamin A as two carrots (738 milligrams to carrots' 713 milligrams) and three times the amount of vitamin C as an orange (164 milligrams to oranges' 46.9 milligrams).[22]

Moringa contains the important minerals chromium and manganese. Chromium is important for blood sugar balance and reducing or eliminating sugar cravings. Manganese is essential for bone formation, healthy joints, reproduction, immune health, and digestion. Moringa also contains more boron than any other plant, a mineral needed for healthy immune function, cognition, and decreased risk of mortality (aka longevity). It's been shown to improve bone density, wound healing, and to even support your body through cancer therapy.[23]

Its range of antioxidants contribute to Moringa being the miracle longevity plant. These antioxidants fight free radicals that can lead to a range of unwanted diseases. And if all that wasn't enough, it also has ample amounts of amino acids and essential omega 3, 6, and 9 fatty acids.

Not surprisingly, Moringa has been studied for its potential benefits with chronic disease. It has shown to be beneficial in "several chronic conditions including hypercholesterolemia, high blood pressure, diabetes, insulin resistance, nonalcoholic liver disease, cancer, and overall inflammation."[24] Whether in prevention or treatment, Moringa is a well-documented ally to bring the body back into a state of health and vitality.

HELPFUL WITH MOOD

Moringa, like Tulsi, supports mood via its mental health and gut-healing properties. It's been used for nervous system ailments in Ayurveda for centuries. Its amino acid profile, particularly tryptophan, supports neurotransmitter function and the feel-good hormone, serotonin. Its antioxidant load helps fight fatigue, mood swings, stress, and depression.

Stress is the first stage of nervous system imbalance and can quickly lead to mental health concerns like anxiety and depression. In a 2015 study, rats that received Moringa leaf extract at 200 milligrams per kilogram of their body weight per day showed significant improvement in behavioral models of depression, a forced swim test, a tail suspension test, and a locomotor activity test. The study's assumed conclusion is that Moringa acts on the same neurotransmitter pathway as SSRIs.[25] The biggest difference is that Moringa doesn't come with the same side effects as SSRIs and instead provides a range of additional benefits to whole-body wellness.

When it comes to digestion, Moringa is so nutrient-dense that it is used as a meal replacement in malnourished communities across the world. It improves digestion, replenishes nutrients, improves growth and performance, and has antioxidant properties. A study comparing Moringa to alfalfa (a well-studied and utilized nutrient-rich herbal medicine) showed that Moringa leaf had a viable impact on all tested metrics, including weight gain and improved liver and spleen index.[26] Beyond its sheer nutrient density, its anti-inflammatory properties have a range of digestion benefits. Moringa has been studied for its ability to treat stomach ulcers, digestive complaints, and colitis with much success.[27]

The combination of brain- and mind-supporting amino acids, antioxidants, minerals, and vitamins make Moringa a promising mood ally. Rather than directly stimulating neurons or classic brain chemicals, it replenishes your body with the nutrients it needs to restore, repair, and perform.

HELPFUL FOR BEAUTY

The connection between Moringa and skin health has a long history. It's been used topically for a range of skin complaints, including psoriasis. Many compounds in Moringa aid in its connection to glowing skin and beauty. Topically, it is highly antibacterial. The leaves are used as a water filtration system because of their ability to kill bacteria such as E. coli and staph from water, and studies examining using Moringa as an alternative to hand soap as an antibacterial agent have shown it is equally effective as traditional soaps.[28] Additionally, the beta-carotene in Moringa can penetrate the skin and boost retinol esters. When these esters are activated, the skin is stimulated to produce new cells that can help fade skin spots and dark pigmentations on the skin. This results in a smoother complexion and helps protect the skin from sun damage. Win-win!

But there's more to beta-carotenes than meets the surface. You may have heard of these as the yellow, orange, and red pigments that give carrots their color. But these famous phytochemicals are produced by plants, algae, bacteria, and fungi, and act as antioxidants. The specific type of carotenoid found in Moringa, beta-carotene, gets converted to vitamin A, a key vitamin for healthy eyesight and vision that has also been linked to clear, acne-free skin.

When your body doesn't have enough vitamin A, your skin produces excess keratin in the hair follicles. Excess keratin means your body has a harder time sloughing off dead skin cells from its follicles, resulting in blockages and acne. Many acne medications now include vitamin A for this reason.[29] To top it off, Moringa has vitamin C, which is clinically proven to have antiaging and anti-pigmentary properties. It also has vitamin B, which is involved in the maintenance of healthy skin cells and often touted as the secret to healthy skin. Therefore, many natural beauty products, either supplements or topicals, use vitamin Bs.

Lastly, fresh Moringa leaves contain vitamin E at concentrations similar to those found in nuts. Vitamin E not only protects the skin against UV radiation (sun damage) and environmental toxins, but also moisturizes the skin, promotes wound healing, and possesses anti-inflammatory properties.[30]

PREPARATION, SOURCING, AND DOSAGE

Moringa leaf can be eaten like many other greens if harvested young, either raw like dandelion or other early spring greens, or cooked in water or oil. Water will bring out its water-soluble vitamins like C and Bs; oil will bring out its fat-soluble vitamins like E.

If you don't live in a tropical climate where there is access to fresh Moringa leaves, dried leaves will also do the trick. They can be used to make an infusion. You can also purchase them powdered or extracted in alcohol (tinctured). The dried powder is the most common form available, along with being the most potent form, as it is the concentrate of the leaves. Store Moringa powder in airtight, waterproof, and lightproof containers. Miron glass or dark amber glass jars are ideal. It will stay good for several months without losing much potency. As soon as the container is opened, use the powder fairly quickly because exposure to air and water can increase the risk of it going bad.[31]

An effective starting dose of dried powder is a half-teaspoon per day. Since this powder packs such a punch, two teaspoons per day is our recommended upper limit. Our body is not able to absorb more than that amount at one time. If using the powder in a capsule, three capsules is usually about quarter of a teaspoon of powder or about 1.5 grams. If using a tincture, 20 to 30 drops (or about one dropperful) per day is an equivalent effective dose. Always choose certified organic Moringa powder that comes from its native climate. This will ensure the highest quality and the leaf just as nature intended.

REAL-LIFE WAYS TO BENEFIT FROM MORINGA

- *For longevity:* Add powder to a morning smoothie or stir into matcha to fuel your day with preventive longevity support.

- *For stress:* Brew leaves into an infusion (tea) and drink as a daily tonic to keep stress at bay.

- *For beauty:* Cook fresh leaves with healthy fats to help your body absorb the fat-soluble beta-carotene for skin health from the inside out. If you don't have access to fresh leaves, sprinkle Moringa powder over cooked rice, roasted veggies, or on top of a savory dish without exposing the powder to heat to keep its plentiful Vitamin C intact.

ASTRAGALUS

Full legal name: *Astragalus membranaceus* from the *Fabaceae* (legume or pea) family

Nicknames: Longevity root, milkvetch, Huang Qi (which means "yellow leader" in Chinese), logoweed, and young man's Ginseng (although not a real Ginseng)

Power hub: Root

Home: Northern and Eastern regions of China, Mongolia, Korea, and the Siberian region of Russia

Energetics: Warm, moist

Helpful with:

1. Longevity
2. Immunity
3. Recovery

Comes with:

- Astragalans I, II, and III
- Astragolosides
- Glucuronic acid
- Cycloastragenol
- Choline and betaine
- Flavones and isoflavones

Common uses: Change of seasons

Best friends: Reishi, Ginseng, Schisandra, Turmeric, Cordyceps, licorice, milk thistle, and nettle seed

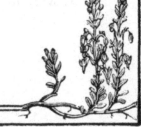

A BRIEF HISTORY: The Root to Recovery

Astragalus has been a powerful tonic for hundreds of years all over Asia. In traditional Mongolian medicine, it is considered one of the 50 fundamental herbs. It's been used for at least two thousand in TCM, where it is listed in the highest class of herbs used in *The Divine Farmer's Classic of Materia Medica*. In China, it is called "yellow leader," partly due to the yellow hue of its root and partly because of its ability to promote the vital force. Astragalus is part of a premier group of herbs called Fu Zheng, meaning to balance or normalize the center. Herbs in this class are known to treat diseases via a twofold mechanism. First, they promote the host's defense mechanism, then they normalize the body's central energy.

In *The Divine Farmer's Classic of Materia Medica*, it's described as being nontoxic and "treats the hundred diseases of small children." It is often referred to as "the young person's Ginseng." This mountainous root gained such praise that it even became an official drug in the modern pharmacopoeia of China, often prescribed for fatigue, loss of appetite, and a general lack of vitality. Traditionally, it was associated with its ability to tonify the kidneys and liver and protect them from further damage.

It wasn't until the 1980s that Astragalus was used in herbal practices in the West. It emerged into Western herbalism after a research hospital in Texas found that the combination of Astragalus and Ligustrum tinctures had a positive benefit on cancerous tumors in mice. Shortly after this, the herbal community quickly jumped on this new (to the West) herb, and it started appearing in almost every herbal company's products and formulation. It is now one of the primary tonic herbs used to bring people back from illness and kickstart their road to recovery. Repairing, rebuilding, and recovery are the key attributes of this root.

HELPFUL WITH LONGEVITY

For thousands of years, Astragalus has been a go-to herb for restoring the life force that brings about a long, fruitful life. It's prescribed as a super tonic of revitalization when the life force is weak, such as in cases of chronic illness.

One of the more unique qualities of Astragalus is its effect on telomeres, the cap-like structures that protect the ends of chromosomes. Telomeres have three primary roles: protect the DNA from damage, ensure that it does not fuse with other chromosomes, and keep DNA at an optimal length.

Telomeres are formed by telomerase, the enzyme that adds the telomere "caps" to the end of DNA strands. Telomeres that are too short go into crisis mode, which can lead to cell death (apoptosis). Telomeres and telomerase are mostly found in fetal tissue, adult germ cells, and tumor cells, and there is interesting research that connects the health of telomeres and telomerase with aging, tumors, and even cancer.[32] This is where the Astragalus root comes in. Astragalus has long been touted as an anti-aging secret because it can protect and even lengthen telomeres.

An essential part of healing tissue is DNA replication, a biological process where a DNA strand gets copied and divided. All organs of our body are formed by tissues. Therefore, tissue health is key to maintain the health of all 78 organs of the body—including the brain, heart, and skin. DNA is in a double helix structure, and in replication, the two strands are separated. From the separation, a new helix is formed from half of the original DNA and half with a newly synthesized strand.

Yet sometimes our cells face a problem. DNA strands in complex cells can't be copied to their very ends. This is where telomeres come in. Every time cells divide, the telomeres get shorter. The shorter each telomere gets, the closer it is to dying. Eventually, the telomere is too short so replication halts and cells die. This is a process of aging on a molecular level. In summation, the shorter your telomeres are, the older your cells are.

On the flip side, longer telomeres tell your body to keep repli-cating and producing more DNA cells. This is anti-aging in action. An extract of Astragalus known as TA-65 has been researched for its anti-aging effects, particularly as it relates to telomerase. While still debated, the compound in Astragalus thought to be respon-sible for this is cycloastragenol. In a 2019 study, Astragalus along-side Gotu Kola was shown to increase telomerase activity 4.3-fold compared to no treatment. It was able to decrease the number of short telomeres and protect cells from DNA damage. On a very literal and physical level, Astragalus is anti-aging.[33]

HELPFUL WITH IMMUNITY

Astragalus's classification as an Adaptogen is primarily due to the way it beneficially affects the immune system. It intensifies white blood cell activity, key components of the immune system. Originally thought to be an action directed by its polysaccha-rides, it's now believed that its triterpenes and other compounds act in concert to produce the immune-stimulating effects.[34]

Astragalus is also antiviral and anti-inflammatory, able to directly fight against pathogens and simultaneously stimulate key immune cells. As a nontoxic herb safe to take daily, Astragalus is particularly potent at helping the immune system *bounce back*. Whether your body is worn down from multiple bouts of illness or one intense sickness, Astragalus's antiviral, anti-inflammatory, and immune restorative actions make it a potent ally. Chinese researchers have been studying Astragalus for years and have repeatedly demonstrated its ability to enhance NK cells and other immune factors.[35]

In TCM, Astragalus is known to strengthen lung Qi, which creates Wei Qi, the protective energy that prevents illness. The stronger the Wei Qi, the more difficult it is to get sick because your system is strong and resilient. In modern-day China, it is still used for this purpose. A key immune enhancer, Astragalus helps prevent ailments ranging from the common cold to even pneumonia and bronchitis.

The key differentiator between Astragalus and many of the other Adaptogens is that it should not be taken during an acute illness, because it can "lock in" the antigen your body is working to fight off. Instead, it is best to take Astragalus immediately after a sickness to help your body to recover and rebuild.

HELPFUL WITH RECOVERY

Astragalus is considered energy-building and stamina-increasing, particularly in cases where the life force is very low and weak. Clinical evidence shows that patients who have undergone extreme therapies have benefitted from using Astragalus during their treatment. After chemotherapy, which greatly reduces the body's natural immune response, people who took Astragalus had reduced side effects, significantly faster recovery, and lived longer. Equally astounding is the research on the main active constituent in Astragalus, astragalosides, having a protective effect on myocardial injuries. A 2005 study on astragalosides at the Research Institute of Cardiovascular Disease found that astragalosides can help with multiple heart issues by reducing calcium overload, enhancing free radical removal, and decreasing oxidative damage to fat cells around the heart muscle.[36] Its high flavonoid content further protects the blood vessels of the heart.

Other research shows Astragalus's anti-fatigue activity.[37] It has even been studied for its ability to enhance growth performance in pigs.[38] This is likely due to its high nutrient content, including various amino acids, vitamins, minerals, and unique phytochemicals.

From its ability to stimulate a weakened immune system to cardiovascular support, Astragalus is a true ally in recovery. The nutrient profile and many phytochemicals still being discovered in the root all work together to help your body revitalize, even in the most extreme illnesses.

PREPARATION, SOURCING, AND DOSAGE

Astragalus can be bought as slices (which need to be extracted in a long hot water decoction), as a dried powder, capsules, or in a tincture. If making a decoction, add two teaspoons of dried sifted root or 10 to 30 grams of flat dried root slices per every 12 ounces of water. Once fully brewed (ideally at least a few hours, up to overnight), drink one to three cups per day. If using a tincture, start with 30 drops (or one dropperful) per day. You can slowly build up to two to three dropperfuls after a few days as your body allows.

In China, the tincture is administered in what they call "Astragalus happy hour." The tincture is prepared with "wine" (50 percent alcohol sake), steeping 10 ounces of Astragalus in two quarts alcohol for one month. It's then suggested to take between 10 milliliters to 60 milliliters up to three times per day.

A crude powder is going to be more potent than the slices of the root, because as more cell surface is exposed, the body is better able to utilize its compounds. Start with two to six grams per day. Begin on the lower end if you are using it as a preventative measure or as a general tonic. Astragalus is one of the safest of the Adaptogens, with no known toxicity.

REAL-LIFE WAYS TO BENEFIT FROM ASTRAGALUS

- *For longevity:* Mix powdered Astragalus in warm water with honey as a daily tonic.

- *For immunity:* Add slices of dried Astragalus to a crockpot and combine with other immune herbs like Reishi and elderberry, vegetables, and mushrooms for an immune-supportive winter broth.

- *For recovery:* Take Astragalus daily in any form the week after getting off any medication to support longevity through its liver-supportive properties.

Evening Hot Chocolate Recipe
for Sleep and Relaxation

Give this decadent and rich hot chocolate recipe a try for a calming and grounding evening. You can also adjust the recipe for desired sweetness by playing with the amount of monk fruit, stevia, or coconut palm sugar.

- 4 squares of organic chocolate made with more than 70 percent real Cacao
- 1 teaspoon of Reishi extract
- 1 teaspoon of Ashwagandha
- Pinch of monk fruit or stevia to taste (coconut palm sugar will also work)
- A few drops of vanilla extract
- Hot foamed plant milk (optional)

Put the chocolate squares in a blender and pour hot water on top. Add the vanilla extract, dry ingredients, and sweetener of choice. Blend for 10 to 15 seconds and open carefully. Alternatively, add hot foamed milk of your choice to turn it into a latte. Enjoy hot!

PART III

YOUR
LIFE ON
ADAPTOGENS

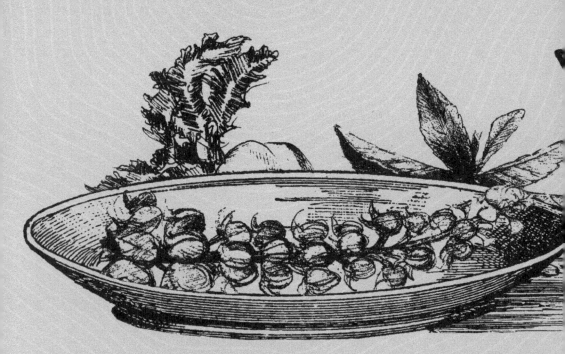

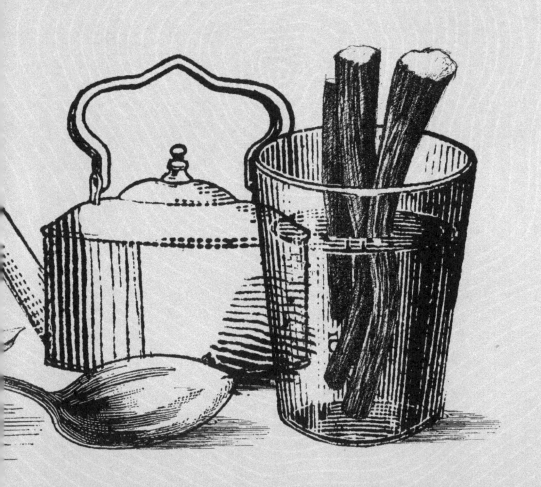

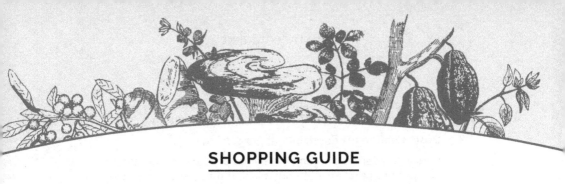

WHAT TO LOOK FOR WHEN BUYING ADAPTOGENS

As you can now see, given the overwhelming demands of modern-day life, Adaptogens are more relevant than ever before. People disappointed in the results of overmedication, decreased nutrition, and poor coping strategies over the last few decades are seeking alternatives. But, with the rise in popularity of natural options to address the stress and symptoms of today, comes both good and bad.

Clever online marketers and other "riffraff" have emerged selling Adaptogens and other superfoods. There have been many scandals (and snake oil salesmen) involved in the sale of such foods. This is especially true with any "super" berry-like acai, products related to weight loss, and sugary or sketchy products like Ashwagandha gummies. In fact, 74 percent of Reishi products sold in the United States are not authentic.[1] So there's often more to quality than meets the eye. As a consumer, you must be extraordinarily careful when new "miracle" foods are marketed aggressively.

Since the marketplace and sourcing constantly changes, it's hard to provide specific "buy this product" type of suggestions. We also want this to be a perennial guide which can stand the test of time. Luckily, there are five key factors that you can check against now and in the future to ensure you are getting a high quality Adaptogen product:

1. **Form.** Ensure the Latin name is listed on the product as well as the form of the product (e.g., leaf, root, fruiting body, etc.).

2. **Dose.** Confirm the dose/amount per serving.

3. **Purity.** Buy certified organic whenever possible. If you can find products that are both organic and third-party lab tested, even better.

4. **Bioavailability.** Buy freshly harvested plants or extracted mushroom products.

5. **Sustainability.** Check the country of origin and information about farming and harvesting practices.

Step 1 is to make sure you have the right form. Are you buying what you want? With Adaptogens, there are *a lot* of fake products out there (don't even get us started on the market for fake Ginseng!). In the supplement facts panel, the words in parentheses after the common name are the true Latin name, aka the botanical name. Look for this to ensure the genus (second word in the Latin name) is correct. This means it should list the full two Latin names, like *Panax ginseng*, as an example. It's not uncommon to see incorrectly labeled products sold in supermarkets. Avoid products that don't disclose the Latin name in their supplement facts panel. If the product has a nutrition facts panel, head to the company's website to confirm details about the ingredient's form and Latin name.

There are also tons of processed Adaptogens. This is especially true when it comes to Cacao or cocoa. Always go for raw and unprocessed Cacao powder. Avoid products that say Dutch processed. With all the functional mushrooms (Chaga, Reishi, Cordyceps, Lion's Mane, and Turkey Tail), avoid products that say mushroom mycelium, mycelial biomass, mushroom powder, full-spectrum, or primordia. These are all marketing ways to avoid the fact that they are not actually using the real mushroom or are only partially using it. According to the FDA, the word mushroom means the fruiting body of the fungi. As such, any product that uses all or part mycelium "should not suggest or imply that the food contains mushrooms on the label."[2] In this book, when we've talked about mushrooms or functional mushrooms, we exclusively are referring to the fruiting bodies of fungi, or the real mushrooms themselves, as defined by both mycologists and the FDA alike.

While consuming mycelium might not be dangerous (unless your diet can't include grains the mycelium is grown on), it means that you're not getting the full benefits from the species. A 2003 paper by the world-famous mycologist Paul Stamets, published in the *International Journal of Medicinal Mushrooms,* shows that myceliated rice only has 2 to 3 percent of active ingredient beta-glucans compared to fruiting bodies at 40 percent. So you must make sure you're truly buying what you are wanting to buy—be it real Cacao, real mushrooms, or real Ginseng. Use our fact boxes in the Adaptogen profiles as a quick reference to ensure you are getting the real deal. Also, avoid overly processed Adaptogens and new or trendy forms that differ from the kind our ancestors have used for millennia.

Once you know that you're getting what you want to get, **Step 2 is that you get the right dose.** Since lying about the genus is technically illegal, creating smoke and mirrors on the dose is often the easiest way shady sellers can misdirect consumers. Technically, the company must honestly provide the dose of Adaptogens per serving, but many food and beverage companies selling Adaptogen drinks or snacks don't.

Even if a company does disclose the dose, there are two things to be careful of: (a) so-called pixie dusting and (b) unclear extraction methods. Pixie dusting refers to a supplement industry method of adding a noneffective dose of an ingredient. A "just so you can say your product includes this" tactic. Most commonly, these products include 20 to 50 such ingredients (think 75 superfoods and Adaptogens in one small scoop of green powder). If you're getting more than 10 Adaptogens in one serving, you're probably getting none.

As a rule of thumb, even with the best extract of anything, you will need to ensure appropriate dosages to reap the benefits. If taking a single dose of one Adaptogen, make sure there is at least 200 to 300 milligrams per serving. If taking a formula with two to five ingredients, look for around 200 to 400 milligrams of each Adaptogen for a total of at least 500 milligrams of total Adaptogens per serving. To summarize, beware of anything that has more than 10 ingredients or less than 100 milligrams per ingredient.

Once you know you're getting what you want, and enough of it, **Step 3 is to make sure it's pure and safe.** Many Adaptogens have the tendency to accumulate toxins from the soil or their growing medium. This can happen for a variety of reasons. With mushrooms, this is part of their role in nature. They help clean and break down toxins (some non-Adaptogenic mushrooms can even difficult waste items like plastics, through a field known as mycoremeditation). Some other Adaptogens are perennial and have plenty of time to concentrate harmful materials.

Ensuring an ingredient is clean and pure requires testing the ingredient for several factors. The key issues to look out for and ensure your ingredient is void of are (i) heavy metals, (ii) pesticides, (iii) mycotoxins, (iv), microbiological issues, and (v) irradiation. There are also tons of layers within each one of these. With heavy metals, the four most-toxic and most-tested heavy metals include arsenic, cadmium, lead, and mercury. Pesticides are a broad group of chemicals that kill insects, fungi, weeds, etc. The insect killers (insecticides) include Cypermethrin, Imidacloprid, and Acetamiprid. The most famous mushroom killer (fungicide) is Carbendazim, and the foremost herb killer (herbicide) is Glyphosate. The latter is better known as Monsanto's Roundup (which is banned in dozens of countries including France, Germany, Italy, and India. Not to mention it also has *thousands* of pending lawsuits against it.). Mycotoxins (i.e., bad fungi) include aflatoxins, ochratoxins, patulin, fusarium, citrinin, and ergot alkaloids. With microbiological issues, you have Escherichia coli, staphylococcus aureus, and more broadly measuring the plate count of microbes. Food irradiation means the ingredients have been exposed to radiation from gamma rays, X-rays, or electron beams. This is typically done to extend the shelf life of a product but can cause dangerous free radicals, so avoid irradiated Adaptogens wherever you can.

So what can you do as a consumer? Buy certified organic products! It doesn't fully guarantee that they won't include heavy metals or that they aren't irradiated. Heck, with USDA organic they could even include some pesticides (wild, right?). But with non-organic products, you will be getting toxins almost 100 percent of the time. Some organic standards are not the best and there is some cheating going on for sure. But maybe that means 5 percent of the time you're building your toxic load, whereas with "conventional" products it can be 100 percent of the time. Plus, with certified organic products you have a *much* higher chance that the company cares about quality from farm to table (soil, harvesting, drying, storage, shipping, and the list goes on). If they don't care about organic agriculture with all the USDA loopholes, then they probably don't care about the deeper stuff.

If a company claims to use organic ingredients but isn't certified, there's a super-high chance it is lying. Why would you pay a huge 30 to 100 percent premium in cost while forfeiting the benefits of having it on your label? Or even bigger red flags are when a product says it is beyond organic, or something like that. Again, high chance of fraud. The actual "beyond organic" is called Demeter, or biodynamic farming, which can still be labeled organic. Wildcrafted ingredients can even be certified organic now, so please stick to this quality standard if possible. It honestly helps expose over 80 percent of the wheat from the chaff.

Now that you have the right stuff, enough of the stuff, and the stuff is clean. Cool! **Step 4 is to make sure it is bioavailable to your body**, which means that you are actually able to absorb it. There are obviously huge differences between different Adaptogens, but generally aim to purchase freshly picked plants and properly extracted mushrooms. Freshness matters if you're not buying extracts (think Goji, Schisandra, Acerola, Moringa, and Gynostemma). Just like with normal herbs and spices, a lot of the quality goes down with exposure to oxygen. In stores, look for products that were produced more recently. There's usually a lot code that includes a month and year.

Another way some companies cheat is with unclear or poor extraction methods. Now, 100 milligrams of good Ashwagandha means a 10:1 ratio of extracted Ashwagandha powder. This means the crude amount of Ashwagandha root (the original amount before it was extracted) weighs one thousand milligrams (or one gram). A higher extract ratio doesn't always mean it's better. It does impact the dose, however.

We always choose extracts that include all active compounds (versus isolated compounds like rosavins from Rhodiola or beta-glucans from functional mushrooms). Legitimate extracts usually range between a 4:1 and 16:1 ratio. The most commonly used ratio is 10:1. We've included some dosage guidance in each Adaptogen's How to Use section. Please use that as your guide.

Next look for recipes made by herbalists, or which mention synergistic formulation. For example, including vitamin C with Adaptogenic mushrooms increases the absorption of the active compounds. Combining black pepper (the key compound for synergy being piperine) with Turmeric increases the absorption of Turmeric's active compound curcumin. Cacao has a synergistic effect with cayenne pepper. And the list goes on. We've included the "Best friends" section in each Adaptogen's profile so you'll know the classic pairings to try.

Step 5 is to always look out for sustainability. Despite common misconceptions, these are a nonissue with most Chaga and Cordyceps products, but can be a real issue with Cacao, Maca, Goji, and Ginseng. Finding this information can be difficult, but generally, we advise you to go to the company's website and see if it has information about the country of origin or a section about sustainability. If the company doesn't disclose either, then assume that it is poorly sourced and/or unsustainable. If they took the time to care about this, then they would probably also take the time to reflect it in their marketing.

Be critical of hyperbole like "best sourcing" or "best ingredients." The world's truly best thing is probably not available commercially to you over the Internet or on a retail shelf, but high-quality certified organic products are. Choosing organic will help ensure our topsoil doesn't get depleted, our forests remain full of fungi, and our Adaptogen farmers get paid enough. Just like the certified organic logo, it gives an indication that people care about the food they make or sell. It shows that they have an eye for details and that they take pride in making something they also want to consume. It can be a solid positive or negative about all things related to quality.

Final word. This shopping guide is the most dire part about this book after all the fireworks about how wonderful Adaptogens are and can be. Don't let this section stop your enthusiasm. While direct-response marketing, get-rich-quick supplement companies, and multilevel marketing are hurting Adaptogens, remember Adaptogens' ancient intent. Adaptogens are sacred. They are here to heal and be magical. You might need to cut through some BS to find the ancient intent, but it's there. Keep searching. Remain critical but not cynical.

WHERE TO BUY ADAPTOGENS

The need for the benefits that come from using Adaptogens is only increasing by the day. As such, we are seeing more and more brands emerge into the Adaptogen space. Now that you know the tips and tricks on how to vet high-quality products, we hope you have the confidence to go out on your own and source high-quality, effective Adaptogens. This section will help you even further to know exactly where you can purchase Adaptogens in their various forms in the marketplace and what red flags to avoid when doing so. It's worth noting that as knowledge of these ingredients grows, the amount of high-quality, mainstream, and affordable options will ideally grow with it.

From in-person locations to online e-tailers, Adaptogens are available across the board. There are some brands that, as of now, will primarily be found in health food stores or specific websites. Others can be found in Costco and on Amazon with a wide range of quality.

If you are an in-person shopper, head to any natural food store like Whole Foods Market, Sprouts Farmers Market, Natural Grocers, or a local co-op in your area. Use our vetting suggestions to choose the best supplement or product. More conventional supermarkets are also catching on to the need for Adaptogens on store shelves. You can find more common Adaptogens like Turmeric, Cacao, and Ashwagandha at Target, Costco, and conventional markets. If you prefer to shop online, the world is truly your oyster. From bigger options like Costco and Amazon to smaller e-tailers like Thrive Market and iHerb, Adaptogens are making themselves known on the World Wide Web (as well as the underground mycelium "wood wide web").

Our favorite supplement companies for Adaptogenic herbs, specifically the plant species, are Gaia Herbs, Herb Pharm, Quantum Nutrition Labs, Organic India, and Wishgarden. Companies like Gaia Herbs can be found in all Whole Foods Markets across the nation, while others like Wishgarden may be a bit more niche to a local pharmacy or health food store (or directly on their website). When it comes to functional mushroom products, our favorites are Four Sigmatic, Real Mushrooms, Mushroom Revival, and Superfeast. All of these brands use mushroom fruiting bodies that have been properly extracted and tested to ensure the cleanest products possible.

If you are ready to dive into using raw materials like Adaptogenic powders or dried whole mushrooms to make your own medicine at home, there are many options available to you. Our favorite online herb stores for bulk materials are Mountain Rose Herbs, Starwest Botanicals, Frontier Co-op, Avena Botanicals, and Omica Organics.

If you are going outside of our top recommendations, there are some major dos and don'ts to be aware of to ensure you are actually getting true Adaptogens in a high-quality form, in the right dose. Essentially, pause before you reach for gummies that claim to have Adaptogens in them from places like Walmart and Costco.

There is a lot of "pixie dusting" on the market. This means brands claiming that there are Adaptogens in a product but are putting in too small of an amount for you to receive any benefits. Watch out for when the name of an Adaptogen appears on a label but is absent from the nutrition facts or supplement facts label. Also watch out for nonorganic Adaptogens. The last thing we want is for you to start taking an Adaptogen to support your health and wind up consuming a supplement full of heavy metals or pesticides instead.

We also suggest avoiding low- or dubious-quality capsules. This is because it's easy to hide poor quality behind the encapsulation. Furthermore, in following ancient traditions, it's believed that the medicine starts in your mouth. This means that by tasting the plant or mushroom, a cascade of reactions takes place in your body. The flavor of the ingredient is the first step to that Adaptogen working in your body. For example, the bitter flavor of certain functional mushrooms automatically signals the liver to start kicking into high gear and increasing its detoxification effects.

All Adaptogens should be tasted whenever possible. This can be done through powders, food-like formulas, tinctures, or the bulk ingredient itself (especially when it comes to Adaptogens like Goji and Cacao). If you do end up with a capsule and want to test to ensure it is high quality, open one up and taste the ingredients inside. This is a great test for mushroom supplement quality. A high-quality product should be dark in color and strong and bitter tasting. If it's sweet or tastes like a graham cracker, that's a red flag that it's not meeting the quality standards of form, dose, purity, bioavailability, or sustainability. Additionally, opening your capsules and tasting what's inside will greatly enhance your body's ability to utilize and recognize the plant or mushroom being consumed.

TOP 10 COMMANDMENTS OF ADAPTOGENS

1. Listen to your body. Bioindividuality is so important when it comes to Adaptogens. Even after you learn about an ingredient, remember that it may affect your body in unique or unexpected ways. Listen to what your body is telling you and either continue or discontinue use based on your own unique experience and needs.

2. Adaptogens are supplemental tools. They should never be used as a replacement for a healthy diet, exercise, good sleep, and general well-being practices. Instead, they should be used as additions to your wellness journey. We never want you to rely on anything to help get through the day. Make sure your underlying needs are met and then use Adaptogens to support your body beyond your basic needs.

3. Always start small. Begin using a new Adaptogen at the lowest end of the dosing recommendation and slowly build up from there, increasing in small increments week by week.

4. For best results, take Adaptogens 30 minutes before food.

5. Always purchase Adaptogens that are certified organic.

6. Functional mushrooms supplements should always meet the following criteria:

    i.   Mushroom fruiting body (aka real mushroom)

    ii. Grown on log, wood, or wild-harvested (exception: Cordyceps, because it is the only Adaptogenic functional mushroom that does not naturally grow on wood; it grows on insects. For humanitarian and sustainability reasons, lab-grown Cordyceps is recommended and often the highest quality you can find.)

    iii. Extracted properly (dual-extract is the gold standard)

    iv. Third-party lab tested

7. Choose Adaptogens from their native countries. (e.g., Ashwagandha from India and Reishi from China).

8. Stay away from capsules if possible. Poor quality or rancid ingredients can hide inside capsules.

9. Taste your Adaptogens. It has often been said that "the medicine starts in your mouth." Essentially, when your body tastes the flavor, a cascade of reactions begins in your body. This allows your body to instantly recognize the ingredient and enhances the functional benefits. If you do purchase

capsules for ease of use, simply open one up, pour the contents on your hand, and taste them.

10. Keep an open mind. New research is constantly being conducted, discoveries are always being made, and Adaptogens will continue to surprise you when used at different times in your life. Stay curious and have fun with them!

CREATING YOUR ROUTINE: A MULTIFACETED APPROACH

The baseline daily routine we recommend is Defend Adaptogens in the morning, Perform Adaptogens in the afternoon, and Restore Adaptogens in the evening. We didn't label them as Morning, Afternoon, and Evening Adaptogens because their versatile nature allows you to take them based on the constantly changing challenges of your daily routine. You could start a lazy Sunday morning with a Restore Adaptogen, but on a weekday morning you may have to jump out of bed to quickly Perform.

Take our guidance as a starting direction to help you get going but remain flexible as much as possible. After all, we're all different and our own situations are constantly changing. Seasons change, stress goes up and down with surprising stimuli, and external obstacles occur. Always listen to your body and trust in the nonspecific balancing power of Adaptogens for your needs.

Prepare for some major surprises once you start using Adaptogens consistently. Once you start using allies like Ashwagandha to sleep better, you may find your performance increases as well. Start taking Lion's Mane for brain power and productivity at work, but don't be surprised if you notice your immune system also starts to improve. Beyond what we call out as the key benefits for each mushroom, remember that *all* Adaptogenic functional mushrooms *also* support gut health and immunity. And don't ignore Defend Adaptogens when you're not sick or particularly concerned with beauty. As you will learn, Adaptogens like Eleuthero are also amazing for performance and Schisandra for long-term health.

The initial descriptions are just a starting point to show the Adaptogens' key benefits on a spectrum. They all share key characteristics, but some are gentler and more nourishing (Tulsi and Reishi), while others are a bit pushier and stimulating (Rhodiola and Ginseng). Always keep in mind that when it comes to Adaptogens, there is much more than meets the eye. These Adaptogens work in mysterious ways.

Even if you have a ton of information and resources about Adaptogens, it can still be challenging to take the first step toward bringing them into your routine. Let's discuss the most common hurdles we hear that hold someone back from beginning their journey with Adaptogens and offer suggestions to help you get started.

Excuse 1: "I don't have enough time to take all these Adaptogens!"

If you're pinched for time, rather than needing to add a new habit or task to your day, we recommend upgrading habits you already have. You can purchase products you are used to taking that have been enhanced with Adaptogens.

Solution 1: Drink it with your coffee: A simple place to start for most is with a morning cup of coffee. Since over 70 percent of Americans drink coffee every day, there are products with real, organic coffee beans plus high-quality Adaptogen extracts.

Solution 2: Eat them as snacks: another quick option is to have Adaptogens as snacks. Costco sells bulk organic Goji berries. Throw a handful in your morning smoothie, breakfast bowl, trail mix, or simply eat them on their own for an Adaptogenic pick-me-up anywhere you go.

Solution 3: Batch prep Adaptogens in an easy-to-use format, like "power balls." If you're pressed for time in the moment but set aside an evening or day of the week to prepare your meals ahead of time, add an Adaptogenic Cacao (aka homemade chocolate) or Adaptogenic power ball recipe to your weekly routine.

Making your own Cacao can be as simple as three ingredients: Cacao powder (make sure to *not* confuse this with the lower quality and more highly processed cocoa powder), Cacao butter, and a sweetener of your choice (maple syrup or honey work great). You can get creative with Cacao by adding other Adaptogens like Maca or Reishi extract to the weekly batch. Keep in your freezer and bite off a chunk whenever you need it.

To make power balls, simply blend nut butter (we love almond butter for this), dates, a pinch of salt, and any powdered Adaptogen extracts. Blend, roll up into balls, and store in an airtight container in the refrigerator or freezer for up to a few weeks.

Excuse 2: "I won't remember to take them!"

If you're terrible at remembering to take any new supplement or vitamin or even have a difficult time purchasing new and unfamiliar products or ingredients, we've got you covered. Some of our favorite ways to get used to bringing Adaptogens on board is to stack Adaptogens on top of our current habits. This is similar to the "pinched for time" category.

Think about the things you already do every day. Do you have some sort of habitual routine in the morning, midday, or in the evening? What can you not wake up without or go to bed without? Almost all of us drink something first thing in the morning and consume something before we hit the hay. Start by noticing your patterns. This may take a few days. Don't be hard on yourself for being forgetful! Simply notice what you reach for at different times of the day. Or think back on your week and notice if there was anything you did multiple times, perhaps even every day. Now get creative with adding Adaptogens to those existing routines. Morning coffee, smoothie, cup of warm water, or something sweet in the evening.

Consider prepping the night before so when you wake up, it's already done for you. The mushrooms are already in your coffee pot, ready to brew. The Adaptogen powder has already been put out on the counter in front of your toaster so you remember to sprinkle a bit of Lion's Mane extract on your avocado toast. Notice your routine, prepare ahead of time, and get creative with adding Adaptogens into each step of your day for seamless, no-thinking-necessary actions. And once you start feeling the benefits, you will surely not forget them (just like many people never forget to have their morning cup of coffee).

Excuse 3: "They're too expensive; I can't afford them!"

If you're ready to start using Adaptogens but are concerned about the price tag, we're here to help. A great option is to look for strong products that will essentially give you the most bang for your buck. Look for bulk options, and pay attention to the total extracted milligrams and price to calculate your price per serving. You can even start with half of the recommended serving, making sure you are still taking an effective dose of at least 500 mg. This will immediately halve the price per serving and still give you a potent starting dose. Product subscriptions and large annual sales (like Black Friday) also offer great value pricing.

Look for other strong products that are offered in bulk, as these typically have high doses for a smaller price tag. You can also start with more commonly available Adaptogens that have a wider distribution and, as such, more competition and a more competitive price. Turmeric is a great option, as it is the most mainstream and widely consumed Adaptogen on the market today.

You can also consider adding some of the "best friends" that are mentioned in each Adaptogen's profile to help ensure that your body will be able to utilize as much as possible from the Adaptogen. Examples include adding black pepper to Turmeric or adding vitamin C–rich foods like rose hips to mushroom products. You can also buy large bags of bulk Adaptogens from places like Mountain Rose Herbs, Starwest Botanicals, and Frontier Co-op for a relatively low cost per serving.

Excuse 4: "I'm sure they'll taste gross, and then I won't take them, so it'll be a waste of money."

If you have a picky palate, don't fret. Several Adaptogens can have a full flavor including bitter or unfamiliar tastes to the common flavors of your day. Don't let this stop you from bringing them into your routine! There are many ways to get creative and still truly enjoy using them. When it comes to bitter Adaptogens like many functional mushrooms, think about combining them with other bitter flavors that you know and love. The two most adored bitter flavors are chocolate and coffee. Adding bitter Adaptogens to your morning cup of Joe or into your hot chocolate or home-made Cacao may truly impress even your most judgmental taste buds. Sneaking a scoop of Adaptogen powder into a smoothie with other more dominant flavors like cinnamon, fruits, and nut butters is another trick. Creating a medicinal broth using functional mushrooms and Adaptogenic roots, especially in colder climates or winter months, can be a delicious treat.

In the world of herbal medicine, corrigents are essentially ingredients that help to improve the flavor of a base ingredient. Honey is one of our favorite corrigents that you can add to your herbal medicine to make it more delicious and easier to consume, as well as to balance its energetics or constitutional actions. The Medical Dictionary defines it as "a drug that modifies or corrects an undesirable or injurious effect of another drug."[1]

You can make an infused honey by adding scoops of Adaptogen extracts into a local, organic honey and then stir into tea or on toast for a sweet, medicinal upgrade to honey. Herbs like cinnamon, licorice, and ginger can also greatly help with the flavor of less desirable–tasting Adaptogens. Consider brewing these herbs into your Adaptogenic decoction or infusion (tea) to enhance the palatability.

There are companies that have made this process simple for you. Nowadays you can find delicious products with potent doses of Adaptogens. You can find everything from mushroom coffees to plant-based protein powders to mushroom Cacao mixes that taste like a delicious mug of European-style hot chocolate.

Excuse 5: "After all of this, I still feel unsure where to start."

If you live in the US, go to the American Herbalist's Guild (AHG) website, www.americanherbalistsguild.com. On the AHG website, click 'Our Members' and then 'Find a Registered Herbalist. If you live in another country, go to Google and search "holistic health care practitioners near me." Or, alternatively, search "herbal practitioners near me." Then find two to five names living near you from those search results. Now, again, search or look up their reviews on Google or Yelp. Try to find someone with many reviews even if one or two are not the best possible. You want someone working actively and with experience of many clients.

Don't find anyone near you? Or don't like their reviews? Alternatively do a similar search but include words like "online consulting." You should be able to find many top herbalists and holistic practitioners who see clients remotely through telemedicine. Some are even a bit cheaper, or you can get more experienced advisors for the same cost.

FINAL WORDS TO GET STARTED

If you have moved beyond all the common reasons that might make it tough for you to start using Adaptogens consistently and you're ready for a full-blown deep dive routine suggestion, let's go! We must preface this section by reminding you that there is not one routine that is best for every person. Instead, remember that the Adaptogens are unique, as is your constantly changing body.

Notice your current symptoms, identify your constitution, and the time of the year or season, and then lean into the Adaptogen(s) best for your current circumstance. Choose an Adaptogen from each of the categories: Defend, Perform, and Restore. Try starting your morning with the Adaptogen in the Defend category to support your baseline vitality for the day. Add a midday Perform Adaptogen to give you the afternoon boost you need to keep going without unhealthy coping strategies. End the day by adding in a Restore Adaptogen, helping you to get to sleep and start the routine over again.

If you are totally new to consuming Adaptogens, don't overdo it! You can still jump into this three-tiered routine system, but make sure you are dosing appropriately. You can also just pick one Adaptogen and start with taking that single ingredient daily. This is called a "simple" in herbal terms and can be a great way to get to know one specific Adaptogen and intimately learn how your body shifts and responds to that plant or mushroom.

Whether you start with one or multiple, be consistent. Building a routine and ensuring you use the Adaptogen consistently will ensure you reap the benefits. Focus on consistency, habit building, and finding a simple way to bring these into your routine for long-term success. Always, always, always start with even less than you think you need, as you can always build up from there.

Regardless of where you are now, meet yourself where you are at. Adaptogens are allies. They are here to support you and help you remember that regardless of how hectic the external or even internal world may seem, you are not alone. You have the help of these ancient species to guide you, heal you, and bring balance and vitality back into the core of your being.

TEST YOUR LEARNINGS:
MINI QUIZ

A) Who is credited for "discovering" the term Adaptogen?

B) What was the first Adaptogen discovered in the U.S.S.R.?

C) Which Adaptogen was used as a currency?

D) Which Adaptogen can help with nerve growth factor (NGF)?

E) Which Adaptogen's nickname translates to "creative forces of the earth"?

F) Which Adaptogen has all the five flavors?

G) Which Ayurvedic body type (dosha) is classified as fire energy?

H) How much dry or crude Adaptogen is in 300 milligrams of a 16:1 extract?

I) Where do saponins get their name from?

J) What are the Top 10 Commandments of Adaptogens?

Know all the right answers?

E-mail book@foursigmatic.com with the correct answers to claim a free prize.

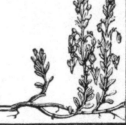

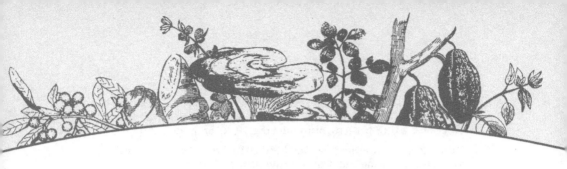

ENDNOTES

INTRODUCTION

1. David Oliver, "Survey: Stress in America Increases for the First Time in 10 Years," Health Buzz, *U.S. News & World Report*, February 15, 2017, https://health.usnews.com/wellness/health-buzz/articles/2017-02-15/survey-stress-in-america-increases-for-the-first-time-in-10-years.

2. Wang et al., "Trends in Consumption of Ultraprocessed Foods Among US Youths Aged 2–19 Years, 1999–2018," *JAMA* 326, no. 6 (2021): 519–530, https://jamanetwork.com/journals/jama/fullarticle/2782866.

3. R. Scheer and D. Moss, "Dirt Poor: Have Fruits and Vegetables Become Less Nutritious?," EarthTalk, *Scientific American*, April 27, 2011, https://www.scientificamerican.com/article/soil-depletion-and-nutrition-loss/.

4. Rochester Epidemiology Project. https://rochesterproject.org/.

PART I

Chapter 1

1. Alexander G Panossian et al., "Evolution of the Adaptogenic Concept from Traditional Use to Medical Systems: Pharmacology of Stress- and Aging-Related Diseases," *Medicinal Research Reviews* (John Wiley and Sons Inc., January 2021), https://www.ncbi.nlm.nih.gov/pmc/articles/PMC7756641/.

2. Liao et al., "A Preliminary Review of Studies on Adaptogens: Comparison of Their Bioactivity in TCM with That of Ginseng-like Herbs Used Worldwide," *Chinese Medicine* 13, no. 57 (November 2018): https://doi.org/10.1186/s13020-018-0214-9.

Chapter 2

1. Tatomir et al., "The Impact of Stress and Glucocorticoids on Memory," *Clujul Medical* 87, no. 1 (January 2014): 3–6, https://www.ncbi.nlm.nih.gov/pmc/articles/PMC4462413/.

2. Coleman et al., "Characterization of Plant-Derived Saponin Natural Products Against Candida Albicans," *ACS Chemical Biology* 5, no. 3 (January 2010): 321–332, https://doi.org/10.1021/cb900243b.

3. K. S. Jyothi and M. Seshagiri, "In-Vitro Activity of Saponins of Bauhinia Purpurea, Madhuca Longifolia, Celastrus Paniculatus and Semecarpus Anacardium on Selected Oral Pathogens," *J Dent (Tehran)* 9, no. 4 (2012): 216–223, https://www.ncbi.nlm.nih.gov/pmc/articles/PMC3536456/.

4. Jayachandran et al., "A Critical Review on the Impacts of β-Glucans on Gut Microbiota and Human Health," *The Journal of Nutritional Biochemistry* 61 (November 2018): 101–110, https://doi.org/10.1016/j.jnutbio.2018.06.010.

5. "Triterpene," ScienceDirect, last modified 2010, https://www.sciencedirect.com/topics/medicine-and-dentistry/triterpene.

6. A. Phaniendra, D. Babu Jestadi, and L. Periyasamy, "Free Radicals: Properties, Sources, Targets, and Their Implication in Various Diseases," *Indian Journal of Clinical Biochemistry* 30, no. 1 (July 2015): 11–26, https://doi.org/10.1007/s12291-014-0446-0.

7. A. N. Panche, A. D. Diwan, and S. R. Chandra, "Flavonoids: An Overview," *Journal of Nutritional Science* 5 (2016): e47, https://doi.org/10.1017/jns.2016.41.

8. Naresh Kumara and Nidhi Goelb, "Phenolic Acids: Natural Versatile Molecules with Promising Therapeutic Applications," *Biotechnology Reports* 24 (December 2019): e00370, https://doi.org/10.1016/j.btre.2019.e00370.

PART II

Chapter 3

For Immunity and Protection

1. Arata et. al, "Continuous Intake of the Chaga Mushroom (Inonotus Obliquus) Aqueous Extract Suppresses Cancer Progression and Maintains Body Temperature in Mice," *Heliyon* 2, no. 5 (May 2016), https://pubmed.ncbi.nlm.nih.gov/27441282/.

2. Hong-Hui Pan et al., "Aqueous Extract from a Chaga Medicinal Mushroom, Inonotus Obliquus (Higher Basidiomycetes), Prevents Herpes Simplex Virus Entry through Inhibition of Viral-Induced Membrane Fusion," *International Journal of Medicinal Mushrooms* 15, no. 1 (2013): 29–38, https://pubmed.ncbi.nlm.nih.gov/23510282/.

3. Shibnev et al., "Antiviral Activity of Aqueous Extracts of the Birch Fungus Inonotus Obliquus on the Human Immunodeficiency Virus," *Vopr Virusol* 60, no. 2 (2015): 35–8, https://pubmed.ncbi.nlm.nih.gov/26182655/.

4. F. Shahzad, D. Anderson, and M. Najafzadeh, "The Antiviral, Anti-Inflammatory Effects of Natural Medicinal Herbs and Mushrooms and SARS-CoV-2 Infection," *Nutrients* 12, no. 9 (August 2020): 2573, https://pubmed.ncbi.nlm.nih.gov/32854262/.

5. S. Jiang, F. Shi, and H. Lin, "Inonotus Obliquus Polysaccharides Induces Apoptosis of Lung Cancer Cells and Alters Energy Metabolism via the LKB1/AMPK Axis," *International Journal of Biological Macromolecules* 151 (May 2020): 1277–1286, https://pubmed.ncbi.nlm.nih.gov/31751687/.

6. Song et al., "Progress on Understanding the Anticancer Mechanisms of Medicinal Mushroom: Inonotus Obliquus," *Asian Pacific Journal of Cancer Prevention* 14, no. 3 (2013): 1571–1578, https://pubmed.ncbi.nlm.nih.gov/23679238/.

7. Yeon-Ran Kim, "Immunomodulatory Activity of the Water Extract from Medicinal Mushroom *Inonotus Obliquus*," *Mycobiology* 33, no. 3 (September 2005): 158–162, https://www.ncbi.nlm.nih.gov/pmc/articles/PMC3774877/.

8. Chen et al., "Purification, Characterization and Biological Activity of a Novel Polysaccharide from Inonotus Obliquus," *International Journal of Biological Macromolecules* 79 (May 2015): 587–94, https://pubmed.ncbi.nlm.nih.gov/26026982/.

9. Han et al., *"Inonotus Obliquus* Polysaccharides Protect against Alzheimer's Disease by Regulating Nrf2 Signaling and Exerting Antioxidative and Antiapoptotic Effects," *International Journal of Biological Macromolecules* 131 (June 2019): 769–778, https://pubmed.ncbi.nlm.nih.gov/30878614/.

10. Han, *"Inonotus Obliquus* Polysaccharides," 769–778.

11. Yun et al., "Inonotus obliquus protects against oxidative stress-induced apoptosis and premature senescence," *Molecules and Cells* 31 (February 2011): 423–429, https://pubmed.ncbi.nlm.nih.gov/21359681/.

12. Zhang et al., "Spatial Structure and Anti-Fatigue of Polysaccharide from Inonotus Obliquus," *International Journal of Biological Macromolecules* 151 (May 2020) 855–860, https://pubmed.ncbi.nlm.nih.gov/32068062/.

13. Yue et al., "Effect of Inonotus Obliquus Polysaccharides on Physical Fatigue in Mice," *Journal of Traditional Chinese Medicine* 35, no. 4 (August 2015): 468–472, https://pubmed.ncbi.nlm.nih.gov/26427119/.

14. "Betulinic Acid," Science Direct, last modified 2022 https://www.sciencedirect.com/topics/pharmacology-toxicology-and-pharmaceutical-science/betulinic-acid.

15. E. A. Dosychev and V. N. Bystrova, "Treatment of Psoriasis with Chaga Fungus Preparations," *Vestnik Dermatologii I Venerologii* (May 1973): 79–83, https://www.Chagatrade.ru/pdfdocs/psoriasis_Chaga.pdf.

16. V. Fabric hood, K. Lipponen, and J. Powerful, "CHAGA (*Inonotus obliquus*)," MetINFO Forest Health, last modified September 2000, http://www.metla.fi/metinfo/metsienterveys/lajit_kansi/inobli-n.htm.

17. E. Kuz'michev, E. Sokolova, and E. Kulikova, "Common Fungal Diseases of Russian Forests," United States Department of Agriculture, Forest Service, https://www.fs.fed.us/nrs/pubs/gtr/gtr_ne279.pdf.

18. Gerontakos et al., "Findings of Russian Literature on the Clinical Application of Eleutherococcus Senticosus (Rupr. & Maxim.): A Narrative Review," *Journal of Ethnopharmacoogy* 278 (October 2021): 114274, https://pubmed.ncbi.nlm.nih.gov/34087398/.

19. B. Bohn, C. T. Nebe, and C. Birr, "Flow-Cytometric Studies with Eleutherococcus Senticosus Extract As an Immunomodulatory Agent," *Arzneimittelforschung* 37, no. 10 (October 1987): 1193–6, https://pubmed.ncbi.nlm.nih.gov/2963645/.

20. Amaryan et. al, "Double-Blind, Placebo-Controlled, Randomized, Pilot Clinical Trial of ImmunoGuard," *Phytomedicine* 10 (2003): 271–285, https://tahomaclinic.com/Private/Articles3/Andrographis/Amaryan%202003%20-%20Andrographis%20%20in%20patients%20with%20Familial%20Mediterranean%20Fever.pdf.

21. Yoshiyuki Kimura and Maho Sumiyoshi, "Effects of Various Eleutherococcus Senticosus Cortex on Swimming Time, Natural Killer Activity and Corticosterone Level in Forced Swimming Stressed Mice," *Journal of Ethnopharmacology* 95, no. 2–3 (December 2004): 447–453, https://pubmed.ncbi.nlm.nih.gov/15507373/.

22. Kuo et al., "The Effect of Eight Weeks of Supplementation with Eleutherococcus Senticosus on Endurance Capacity and Metabolism in Human," *The Chinese Journal of Physiology* 53, no. 2 (April 2010): 105–11, https://pubmed.ncbi.nlm.nih.gov/21793317/.

23. "Siberian Ginseng, Eleuthero (Eleutherococcus senticosus/ Acanthopanax senticosus)," The Association for the Advancement of Restorative Medicine (AARM), last modified 2022, https://restorativemedicine.org/library/monographs/Eleuthero/#sdendnote8sym.

24. Bai et al., "Active Components from Siberian Ginseng (Eleutherococcus Senticosus) for Protection of Amyloid β(25-35)-Induced Neuritic Atrophy in Cultured Rat Cortical Neurons," *Journal of Natural Medicines* 65 (2011): 417–423, https://pubmed.ncbi.nlm.nih.gov/21301979/.

25. Tohda et al., "Inhibitory Effects of Eleutherococcus Senticosus Extracts on Amyloid Beta(25-35)-Induced Neuritic Atrophy and Synaptic Loss," *Journal of Pharmacological Sciences* 107, no. 3 (2008): 329–339, https://pubmed.ncbi.nlm.nih.gov/18612196/.

26. Zhang et al., "Combination of Geniposide and Eleutheroside B Exerts Antidepressant-like Effect on Lipopolysaccharide-Induced Depression Mice Model," *Chinese Journal of Integrative Medicine* 27 (July 2021): 534–541, https://pubmed.ncbi.nlm.nih.gov/31784933/.

27. Jin et al., "Anti-Depressant Effects of Aqueous Extract from Acanthopanax Senticosus in Mice," *Phytotherapy Research* 27, no. 12 (December 2013): 534–541, https://www.researchgate.net/publication/235650246_Anti-depressant_Effects_of_Aqueous_Extract_from_Acanthopanax_senticosus_in_Mice.

28. Soya et al., "Extract from Acanthopanax Senticosus Harms (Siberian Ginseng) Activates NTS and SON/PVN in the Rat Brain," *Bioscience, Biotechnology & Biochemistry* 72, no. 9 (September 2008), 2476–2480, https://pubmed.ncbi.nlm.nih.gov/18776662/.

29. "Medicinal Mushrooms (PDQ®)–Health Professional Version," National Cancer Institute, last modified July 14, 2021, https://www.cancer.gov/about-cancer/treatment/cam/hp/mushrooms-pdq.

30. E. Wong, F. Cheng, and C. Leung, "Efficacy of Yun Zhi (Coriolus Versicolor) on Survival in Cancer Patients: Systematic Review and Meta-Analysis," *Recent Patents on Inflammation & Allergy Drug Discovery* 6, no. 1 (2012): 78–87, https://pubmed.ncbi.nlm.nih.gov/22185453/.

31. Ito et al., "Correlation Between Efficacy of PSK Postoperative Adjuvant Immunochemotherapy for Gastric Cancer and Expression of MHC Class I," *Experimental and Therapeutic Medicine* 3, no. 6 (April 2012): 925–930, https://www.ncbi.nlm.nih.gov/pmc/articles/PMC3438816/.

32. Jeong et al., "Macrophage-Stimulating Activity of Polysaccharides Extracted from Fruiting Bodies of Coriolus versicolor (Turkey Tail Mushroom)," *Journal of Medicinal Food* 9, no. 2 (February 2006): 175–81, https://www.researchgate.net/publication/6963234_Macrophage-Stimulating_Activity_of_Polysaccharides_Extracted_from_Fruiting_Bodies_of_Coriolus_versicolor_Turkey_Tail_Mushroom.

33. Pallav et al., "Effects of Polysaccharopeptide from Trametes Versicolor and Amoxicillin on the Gut Microbiome of Healthy Volunteers: A Randomized Clinical Trial," *Gut Microbes* 5, no. 4 (July 2014): 458–467, https://pubmed.ncbi.nlm.nih.gov/25006989/.

34. W. Scheppach, "Effects of Short Chain Fatty Acids on Gut Morphology and Function," *Gut* 35, no. 1 (January 1994): S35–S38, https://www.ncbi.nlm.nih.gov/pmc/articles/PMC1378144/.

35. Chambers et al., "Role of Gut Microbiota-Generated Short-Chain Fatty Acids in Metabolic and Cardiovascular Health," *Current Nutrition Reports* 7 (September 2018): 198–206, https://link.springer.com/article/10.1007/s13668-018-0248-8.

36. Yu et al., "*Trametes Versicolor* Extract Modifies Human Fecal Microbiota Composition *in Vitro*," *Plant Foods for Human Nutrition* 68 (February 2013): 107–112, https://pubmed.ncbi.nlm.nih.gov/23435630/.

37. Pallav et al., "Effects of Polysaccharopeptide," 458–467.

38. Mark et al., "Vitamin D Promotes Protein Homeostasis and Longevity via the Stress Response Pathway Genes skn-1, ire-1, and xbp-1," *Cell Reports* 17, no. 5 (October 2016): 1227–1237, https://pubmed.ncbi.nlm.nih.gov/27783938/.

39. Janjušević et al., "The Lignicolous Fungus *Trametes Versicolor* (L.) Lloyd (1920): A Promising Natural Source of Antiradical and AChE Inhibitory Agents," *Journal of Enzyme Inhibition and Medical Chemistry* 32, no. 1 (January 2017): 355–362, https://www.ncbi.nlm.nih.gov/pmc/articles/PMC6010034/.

40. Francisco Pérez-Cano and Margarida Castell, "Flavonoids, Inflammation and Immune System," *Nutrients* 8, no. 10 (October 2016): 659, https://www.ncbi.nlm.nih.gov/pmc/articles/PMC5084045/.

For Beauty and Skin

1. "History of Turmeric - An In Depth Look at How This Golden Spice Became So Powerful," Me First Living, last modified 2022, https://mefirstliving.com/pages/history-of-Turmeric.

2. Al. Vaughn, A. Branum, and R. Sivamani, "Effects of Turmeric (Curcuma longa) on Skin Health: A Systematic Review of the Clinical Evidence," *Phytotherapy Research* 30, no. 8 (May 2016): 1243–1264, https://pubmed.ncbi.nlm.nih.gov/27213821/.

3. Aggarwal et al., "Curcumin: The Indian Solid Gold," *Advances in Experimental Medicine and Biology* 595 (2007): 1–75, https://pubmed.ncbi.nlm.nih.gov/17569205/.

4. Ganesh Jagetia and Bharat Aggarwal, "'Spicing Up' of the Immune System by Curcumin," *Journal of Clinical Immunology* 27 (January 2007): 19–35, https://pubmed.ncbi.nlm.nih.gov/17211725/.

5. Thimmulappa et al., "Antiviral and Immunomodulatory Activity of Curcumin: A Case for Prophylactic Therapy for COVID-19," *Heliyon* 7, no. 2 (February 2021): e06350, https://pubmed.ncbi.nlm.nih.gov/33655086/.

6. Biswas et al., "Curcumin protects DNA damage in a chronically arsenic-exposed population of West Bengal," *Human & Experimental Toxicology* 29, no. 6 (January 2010): 513–24, https://pubmed.ncbi.nlm.nih.gov/20056736/.

7. Bharat Aggarwal and Bokyung Sung, "Pharmacological basis for the role of curcumin in chronic diseases: an age-old spice with modern targets," *Trends in Pharmacological Sciences* 30, no. 2 (February 2009): P85–94, https://pubmed.ncbi.nlm.nih.gov/19110321/.

8. Nita Chainani-Wu, "Safety and Anti-Inflammatory Activity of Curcumin: A Component of Tumeric (Curcuma longa)," *The Journal of Alternative and Complementary Medicine* 9, no. 1 (July 2004): 161–8, https://pubmed.ncbi.nlm.nih.gov/12676044/.

9. G Shoba et al., "Influence of Piperine on the Pharmacokinetics of Curcumin in Animals and Human Volunteers," *Planta medica* 64(4), 353–356: (May 1998), https://pubmed.ncbi.nlm.nih.gov/9619120/.

10. Chainani-Wu, "Safety and Anti-Inflammatory Activity of Curcumin: A Component of Tumeric (Curcuma longa)," 161–8.

11. Ma et al., "Goji Berries as a Potential Natural Antioxidant Medicine: An Insight into Their Molecular Mechanisms of Action," *Oxidative Medicine and Cellular Longevity* 2019 (January 2019): 2437397, https://www.ncbi.nlm.nih.gov/pmc/articles/PMC6343173/.

12. H. Amagase, B. Sun, and C. Borek, "*Lycium Barbarum* (Goji) Juice Improves In Vivo Antioxidant Biomarkers in Serum of Healthy Adults," *Nutrition Research* 29, no. 1 (January 2009): 19–25, https://pubmed.ncbi.nlm.nih.gov/19185773/.

13. "Adult Growth Hormone Deficiency," Cedars Sinai, last updated 2021, https://www.cedars-sinai.org/health-library/diseases-and-conditions/a/adult-growth-hormone-deficiency.html.

14. H. Amagase, B. Sun, and D. Nance, "Immunomodulatory Effects of a Standardized *Lycium Barbarum* Fruit Juice in Chinese Older Healthy Human Subjects," *Journal of Medicinal Food* 12, no. 5 (October 2009): 1159–65, https://pubmed.ncbi.nlm.nih.gov/19857084/.

15. Moon et al., "Administration of Goji (*Lycium Chinense* Mill.) Extracts Improves Erectile Function in Old Aged Rat Model," *The World Journal of Men's Health* 35, no. 1 (April 2017): 43–50, https://pubmed.ncbi.nlm.nih.gov/28064475/.

16. Yuan et al., "The Traditional Medicine and Modern Medicine from Natural Products, *Molecules* 21, no. 5 (May 2016): 559, https://www.ncbi.nlm.nih.gov/pmc/articles/PMC6273146/.

17. Nowak et al., "Potential of *Schisandra Chinensis* (Turcz.) Baill. in Human Health and Nutrition: A Review of Current Knowledge and Therapeutic Perspectives," *Nutrients* 11, no. 2 (February 2019): 333, https://www.ncbi.nlm.nih.gov/pmc/articles/PMC6412213/.

18. Alexander Panossian and Georg Wikman, "Effects of Adaptogens on the Central Nervous System and the Molecular Mechanisms Associated with Their Stress—Protective Activity," *Pharmaceuticals* 3, no. 1 (January 2010): 188–224, https://www.ncbi.nlm.nih.gov/pmc/articles/PMC3991026/.

19. Kam-Ming Ko and Po-Yee Chiu, "Biochemical Basis of the 'Qi-invigorating' Action of Schisandra Berry (Wu-Wei-Zi) in Chinese Medicine," *The American Journal of Chinese Medicine* 34, no. 2 (2006): 171–6, https://pubmed.ncbi.nlm.nih.gov/16552829/.

20. Ko et al., "Biochemical Basis," 171–6.

21. Panossian et al., "Effects of Heavy Physical Exercise and Adaptogens on Nitric Oxide Content in Human Saliva," *Phytomedicine* 6, no. 1 (March 1999): 17–26, https://pubmed.ncbi.nlm.nih.gov/10228607/.

22. Panossian et al., "Effects of Adaptogens," 188–224.

23. Wakabayashi et al., "Inhibition of LPS-stimulated NO production in mouse macrophage-like cells by Barbados cherry, a fruit of Malpighia emarginata DC," *Anticancer Research* 23, no. 4 (July–August 2003): 3237-41, https://pubmed.ncbi.nlm.nih.gov/12926058/.

24. Anand Prakash and Revathy Baskaran, "Acerola, an Untapped Functional Superfruit: A Review on Latest Frontiers," *Journal of Food Science and Technology* 55, no. 9 (September 2018): 3373–3384, https://pubmed.ncbi.nlm.nih.gov/30150795/.

25. Prakash et al., "Acerola, an Untapped Functional Superfruit," 3373–3384.

26. Prakash et al., "Acerola, an Untapped Functional Superfruit," 3373–3384.

27. Klosterhoff et al., "Anti-Fatigue Activity of an Arabinan-Rich Pectin from Acerola (Malpighia Emarginata)," *International Journal of Biological Macromolecules* 109, no. 1 (April 2018): 1147–1153, https://pubmed.ncbi.nlm.nih.gov/29157904/.

Chapter 4

For Energy and Performance

1. Dr. Stephen Fulder, *The Ginseng Book, Nature's Ancient Healer* (New York: Avery, 1996).

2. Bach et al., "Efficacy of Ginseng Supplements on Fatigue and Physical Performance: A Meta-Analysis," *Journal of Korean Medical Science* 31, no. 12 (December 2016): 1879–1886, https://pubmed.ncbi.nlm.nih.gov/27822924/.

3. Jin et al., "Clinical and Preclinical Systematic Review of *Panax Ginseng* C. A. Mey and Its Compounds for Fatigue," *Frontiers in Pharmacology* 11 (July 2020): 1031, https://pubmed.ncbi.nlm.nih.gov/32765262/.

4. Kim et al., "Korean Red Ginseng for Cancer-Related Fatigue in Colorectal Cancer Patients with Chemotherapy: A Randomised Phase III Trial," *European Journal of Cancer* 130 (Mary 2020): 51–62, https://www.sciencedirect.com/science/article/pii/S0959804920300721.

5. Kar Wah Leung and Alice St Wong, "Ginseng and Male Reproductive Function," *Spermatogenesis* 3, no. 3 (July 2013): e26391, https://pubmed.ncbi.nlm.nih.gov/24381805/.

6. Hong et al., "A Double-Blind Crossover Study Evaluating the Efficacy of Korean Red Ginseng in Patients with Erectile Dysfunction: A Preliminary Report," *Journal of Urology* 168, no. 5 (November 2002): 2070–3, https://pubmed.ncbi.nlm.nih.gov/12394711/.

7. Oh et al., "Effects of Korean Red Ginseng on Sexual Arousal in Menopausal Women: Placebo-Controlled, Double-Blind Crossover Clinical Study," *The Journal of Sexual Medicine* 7, no. 4, part 1 (April 2010): 1469–77, https://pubmed.ncbi.nlm.nih.gov/20141583/.

8. Henrik Sørensen and Jesper Sonne, "A Double-Masked Study of the Effects of Ginseng on Cognitive Functions," *Current Therapeutic Research* 57, no. 12 (December 1996): 959–968, https://www.sciencedirect.com/science/article/abs/pii/S0011393X96801147.

9. D. Kennedy, A. Scholey, and K. Wesnes, "Modulation of Cognition and Mood Following Administration of Single Doses of Ginkgo Biloba, Ginseng, and a Ginkgo/Ginseng Combination to Healthy Young Adults," *Physiology & Behavior* 75, no. 5 (April 2002): 739–751, https://pubmed.ncbi.nlm.nih.gov/12020739/.

10. So et al., "Red Ginseng Monograph," *Journal of Ginseng Research* 42, no. 4 (October 2018): 549–561, https://www.ncbi.nlm.nih.gov/pmc/articles/PMC6190493/.

11. "The Chemical Constituents and Pharmacological Actions of Cordyceps Sinesis," *Evidence-Based Complementary and Alternative Medicine* 2015, no. 2 (April 2015): 1–12, https://www.researchgate.net/publication/275724177_The_Chemical_Constituents_and_Pharmacological_Actions_of_Cordyceps_sinensis.

12. M. Cleaver, and J. Holliday. "On the Trail of the Yak: Ancient Cordyceps in the Modern World," *Earthpulse* (June 2004). https://www.earthpulse.com/cordyceps_inc/cordyceps_story.pdf.

13. Rev M.J. Berkeley, "On Entomogenous Sphaeriae," *The London Journal of Botany* 1843, no. 2 (1843): 205-212. http://cordyceps.us/files/Berkeley_1843_Entomogenous_Sphaeriae.pdf

14. X. Yi, H. Xi-zhen, and Z. Jia-shi, "Randomized Double-Blind Placebo-Controlled Clinical Trial and Assessment of Fermentation Product of Cordyceps Sinesis (Cs-4) in Enhancing Aerobic Capacity and Respiratory Function of the Healthy Elderly Volunteers," *Chinese Journal of Integrative Medicine* 10 (September 2004): 187–192, https://link.springer.com/article/10.1007/BF02836405.

15. Yan-Feng Xu, "Effect of Polysaccharide from *Cordyceps Militaris* (Ascomycetes) on Physical Fatigue Induced by Forced Swimming," *International Journal of Medicinal Mushrooms* 18, no. 12 (2016): 1083–1092, https://pubmed.ncbi.nlm.nih.gov/28094746/.

16. Michael Tierra and David Frawley, *Planetary Herbology: An Integration of Western Herbs into the Traditional Chinese and Ayurvedis Systems* (NA: Lotus Press, 1992).

17. Chen et al., "Effect of Cs-4 (*Cordyceps Sinensis*) on Exercise Performance in Healthy Older Subjects: A Double-Blind, Placebo-Controlled Trial," *The Journal of Alternative and Complementary Medicine* 16, no, 5 (November 2010): 585–590, https://files.achs.edu/course_pdfs/herb504_effect_cs_4_exercise_performance.pdf.

18. Huang et al., "Upregulation of Steroidogenic Enzymes and Ovarian 17β-Estradiol in Human Granulosa-Lutein Cells by *Cordyceps Sinensis* Mycelium," *Biology of Reproduction* 70, 5 (May 2004): 1358–1364, https://academic.oup.com/biolreprod/article/70/5/1358/2712670.

19. Kopalli et al., "Cordycepin, an Active Constituent of Nutrient Powerhouse and Potential Medicinal Mushroom *Cordyceps Militaris* Linn., Ameliorates Age-Related Testicular Dysfunction in Rats," *Nutrients* 11, no. 4 (April 2019): 906, https://pubmed.ncbi.nlm.nih.gov/31018574/.

20. Lin et al., "Improvement of Sperm Production in Subfertile Boars by *Cordyceps Militaris* Supplement," *The American Journal of Chinese Medicine* 35, no. 4 (2007): 631–41, https://pubmed.ncbi.nlm.nih.gov/17708629/.

21. Stone et al., "A Pilot Investigation into the Effect of Maca Supplementation on Physical Activity and Sexual Desire in Sportsmen," *Journal of Ethnopharmacology* 126, no. 3 (December 2009): 574–576, https://pubmed.ncbi.nlm.nih.gov/19781622/.

22. Gonzales et al., "Lepidium Meyenii (Maca) Improved Semen Parameters in Adult Men," *Asian Journal of Andrology* 3, no. 4 (December 2001): 301–3, https://pubmed.ncbi.nlm.nih.gov/11753476/.

23. Stojanovska et al., "Maca Reduces Blood Pressure and Depression, in a Pilot Study in Postmenopausal Women," *Climacteric* 18, no. 1 (June 2014): 1–26, https://www.researchgate.net/publication/263131157_Maca_reduces_blood_pressure_and_depression_in_a_pilot_study_in_postmenopausal_women.

24. Chen et al., "Diary L-Arginine Supplementation Improves Semen Quality and Libido of Boars Under High Ambient Temperature," *Animal* 12, no. 8 (2018): 1611–1620, https://pubmed.ncbi.nlm.nih.gov/29198215/.

25. "Maca's Inner Secrets," Medicine Hunter, last modified 2022, http://www.medicinehunter.com/Macas-inner-secrets.

26. Lee et al., "The Use of Maca (*Lepidium Meyenii*) to Improve Semen Quality: A Systematic Review," *Maturitas* 92 (October 2016): 64–9, https://pubmed.ncbi.nlm.nih.gov/27621241/.

27. Gonzales et al., "Effect of *Lepidium Meyenii* (Maca), a Root with Aphrodisiac and Fertility-Enhancing Properties, on Serum Reproductive Hormone Levels in Adult Healthy Men," Course Hero, last accessed February 2022, https://www.coursehero.com/file/91835873/Effect-of-Lepidium-meyenii-Maca-a-root-with-aphrodisiac-and-fertility-enhancing-properties-on-se/.

28. Zenico et al., "Subjective Effects of *Lepidium Meyenii* (Maca) Extract on Well-Being and Sexual Performances in Patients with Mild Erectile Dysfunction:

A Randomised, Double-Blind Clinical Trial," *Andrologia* 41, no. 2 (February 2009): 95–99, https://pubmed.ncbi.nlm.nih.gov/19260845/.

29. Dording et al., "A Double-Blind, Randomized, Pilot Dose-Finding Study of Maca Root (*L. Meyenii*) for the Management of SSRI-Induced Sexual Dysfunction," *CNS Neuroscience & Therapeutics* 14, no. 3 (August 2008): 182–191, https://pubmed.ncbi.nlm.nih.gov/18801111/.

30. Xia et al., "Simultaneous Determination of Macaenes and Macamides in Maca Using an HPLC Method and Analysis Using a Chemometric Method (HCA) to Distinguish Maca Origin," *Revista Brasileira de Farmacognosia* 29, no. 6 (November–December 2019): 702–9, https://www.sciencedirect.com/science/article/pii/S0102695X18307270.

For Brain and Focus

1. Mori et al., "Improving Effects of the Mushroom Yamabushitake (*Hericium Erinaceus*) on Mild Cognitive Impairment: A Double-Blind Placebo-Controlled Clinical Trial," *Phytotherapy Research* 23, no. 3 (March 2009): 367–72, https://www.researchgate.net/publication/23308681_Improving_Effects_of_the_Mushroom_Yamabushitake_Hericium_erinaceus_on_Mild_Cognitive_Impairment_A_Double-blind_Placebo-controlled_Clinical_Trial.

2. Wong et al., "Peripheral Nerve Regeneration Following Crush Injury to Rat Peroneal Nerve by Aqueous Extract of Medicinal Mushroom *Hericium Erinaceus* (Bull.: Fr) Pers. (Aphyllophoromycetideae)," *Evidence Based Complementary and Alternative Medicine* 2011 (2011): 580752, https://www.ncbi.nlm.nih.gov/pmc/articles/PMC3176599/.

3. Zhang, et al., "The Neuroprotective Properties of *Hericium Erinaceus* in Glutamate-Damaged Differentiated PC12 Cells and an Alzheimer's Disease Mouse Model," *International Journal of Molecular Sciences* 17, no. 11 (November 2016): 1810, https://www.ncbi.nlm.nih.gov/pmc/articles/PMC5133811/.

4. Lampariello et al., "The Magic Velvet Bean of *Mucuna Pruriens*," *Journal of Traditional and Complementary Medicine* 2, no. 4 (October–December 2012): 331–39, https://www.ncbi.nlm.nih.gov/pmc/articles/PMC3942911/.

5. Shukla et al., "Mucuna Pruriens Reduces Stress and Improves the Quality of Semen in Infertile Men," *Evidence-Based Complementary and Alternative Medicine* 7, no. 1 (March 2010): 137–44, https://pubmed.ncbi.nlm.nih.gov/18955292/.

6. Divya et al., "The Traditional Uses and Pharmacological Activities of *Mucuna Pruriens* (L)DC: A Comprehensive Review," *Indo American Journal of Pharmaceutical Research* (2017): 7516–7525, https://www.academia.edu/31318788/THE_TRADITIONAL_USES_AND_PHARMACOLOGICAL_ACTIVITIES_OF_MUCUNA_PRURIENS_L_DC_A_COMPREHENSIVE_REVIEW.

7. Amro et al., "The Potential Role of Herbal Products in the Treatment of Parkinson's Disease," *Clinical Therapeutics* 169, no. 1 (January–February 2018): e23–e33, https://pubmed.ncbi.nlm.nih.gov/29446788/.

8. K. Gohil, J. Patel, and A. Gajjar, "Pharmacological Review on *Centella Asiatica*: A Potential Herbal Cure-All," *Indian Journal of Pharmaceutical*

Sciences 72, no. 5 (September 2010): 546–54, https://pubmed.ncbi.nlm.nih.gov/21694984/.

9. Gray et al., *"Centella Asiatica*—Phytochemistry and Mechanisms of Neuroprotection and Cognitive Enhancement," *Phytochemistry Reviews* 17, no. 1 (February 2018): 161–194, https://pubmed.ncbi.nlm.nih.gov/31736679/.

10. Wu et al., "Oleanane- and Ursane-Type Triterpene Saponins from *Centella Asiatica* Exhibit Neuroprotective Effects," *Journal of Agricultural and Food Chemistry* 1, no. 68 (July 2020): 6977–6986, https://pubmed.ncbi.nlm.nih.gov/32502339/.

11. "Triterpenoid Saponin," ScienceDirect, last modified 2022, https://www.sciencedirect.com/topics/agricultural-and-biological-sciences/triterpenoid-saponin.

12. H. Zhao, R. Sapolsky, and G. Steinberg, "Phosphoinositide-3-Kinase/Akt Survival Signal Pathways Are Implicated in Neuronal Survival After Stroke," *Molecular Neurobiology* 34, no. 3 (December 2006): 249–70, https://pubmed.ncbi.nlm.nih.gov/17308356/.

13. Bradwejn et al., "A Double-Blind, Placebo-Controlled study on the Effects of Gotu Kola (*Centella Asiatica*) on Acoustic Startle Response in Healthy Subjects," *Journal of Clinical Psychopharmacology* 20, no. 6 (December 2000): 680–4, https://pubmed.ncbi.nlm.nih.gov/11106141/.

14. Jana et al., "A Clinical Study on the Management of Generalized Anxiety Disorder with *Centella Asiatica*," *Nepal Medical College Journal* 12, no. 1 (March 2010): 8–11, https://www.researchgate.net/publication/45459786_A_clinical_study_on_the_management_of_generalized_anxiety_disorder_with_Centella_asiatica.

15. Marimuthu et al., "Emerging Role of *Centella Asiatica* in Improving Age-Related Neurological Antioxidant Status," *Experimental Gerontology* 40, no. 8–9 (August 2005): 707–15, https://www.researchgate.net/publication/7717875_Emerging_role_of_Centella_asiatica_in_improving_age-related_neurological_antioxidant_status.

16. Jacinda James and Ian Dubery, "Pentacyclic Triterpenoids from the Medicinal Herb, *Centella Asiatica* (L.) Urban," *Molecules* 14, no. 10 (October 2009): 3922–41, https://pubmed.ncbi.nlm.nih.gov/19924039/.

17. Tsoukalas et al., "Discovery of Potent Telomerase Activators: Unfolding New Therapeutic and Anti-Aging Perspectives," *Molecular Medicine Reports* 20, no. 4 (October 2019): 3701–3708, https://www.ncbi.nlm.nih.gov/pmc/articles/PMC6755196/.

18. Mao et al., "Rhodiola Rosea versus Setraline for Major Depressive Disorder: A Randomized Placebo-Controlled Trial," *Phytomedicine* 22, no. 3 (March 2015): 394–399, https://www.ncbi.nlm.nih.gov/pmc/articles/PMC4385215/.

19. "Comparing Rhodiola Rosea Extracts: Rosavins vs. Salidroside," Nootropics Depot, last modified on June 14, 2018, https://nootropicsdepot.com/articles/comparing-Rhodiola-rosea-extracts-rosavins-vs-salidroside/.

20. De Bock et al., "Acute Rhodiola Rosea Intake Can Improve Endurance Exercise Performance," *International Journal of Sport Nutrition and Exercise Metabolism* 14, no. 3 (June 2004): 298–307, https://pubmed.ncbi.nlm.nih.gov/15256690/.

21. Committee on Herbal Medicine Products (HMPC), "Community Herbal Monograph on *Rhodiola Rosea* L., Rhizoma et Radix," last modified on March 17, 2012, https://www.ema.europa.eu/en/documents/herbal-monograph/final-community-herbal-monograph-Rhodiola-rosea-first-version_en.pdf.

22. M. Cropley, A. Banks, and J. Boyle, "The Effects of *Rhodiola Rosea* L. Extract on Anxiety, Stress, Cognition and Other Mood Symptoms," *Phytotherapy Research* 20, no. 4 (October 2019): 3701–3708, https://pubmed.ncbi.nlm.nih.gov/26502953/.

Chapter 5

For Stress and Mood

1. Singh et al., "An Overview of Ashwagandha: A Rasayana (Rejuvenator) of Ayurveda," *The African Journal of Traditional, Complementary and Alternative Medicine* 8, no. 5 Suppl (July 2011): 208–213, https://www.ncbi.nlm.nih.gov/pmc/articles/PMC3252722/.

2. K. Chandrasekhar, J. Kapoor, and S. Anishetty, "A Prospective, Randomized Double-Blind, Placebo-Controlled Study of Safety and Efficacy of a High-Concentration Full-Spectrum Extract of *Ashwagandha* Root in Reducing Stress and Anxiety in Adults," *Indian Journal of Psychological Medicine* 34, no. 3 (July–September 2012): 255–262, https://www.ncbi.nlm.nih.gov/pmc/articles/PMC3573577/.

3. Auddy et al., "A Standardized *Withania Somnifera* Extract Significantly Reduces Stress-Related Parameters in Chronically Stressed Humans: A Double-Blind, Randomized, Placebo-Controlled Study," *JANA* 11, no. 1 (2008): 50–56, https://blog.priceplow.com/wp-content/uploads/2014/08/withania_review.pdf.

4. "Ashwagandha for Liver Health and Detox: 5 Proven Benefits," Curejoy, last modified September 26, 2016, https://curejoy.com/content/take-Ashwagandha-liver/.

5. T. Kuboyama, C. Tohda, and K. Komatsu, "Effects of Ashwagandha (Roots of Withania Somnifera) on Neurodegenerative Diseases," *Biological and Pharmaceutical Bulletin* 37, no. 6 (2014): 892–7, https://pubmed.ncbi.nlm.nih.gov/24882401/.

6. S. Dubey, M. Kallubai, and R. Subramanyam, "Improving the Inhibition of β-amyloid Aggregation by Withanolide and Withanoside Derivatives," *International Journal of Biological Macromolecules* 173 (March 2021): 56–65, https://pubmed.ncbi.nlm.nih.gov/33465364/.

7. D. Choudhary, S. Bhattacharyya, and S. Bose, "Efficacy and Safety of Ashwagandha (Withania Somnifera (L.) Dunal) Root Extract in Improving Memory and Cognitive Functions," *Journal of Dietary Supplements* 14, no. 6 (November 2017): 599–612, https://pubmed.ncbi.nlm.nih.gov/28471731/.

8. Sukanya Soksawatmakhin and Wijit Boonyahotra, "Preliminary Study of the Applications of *Ganoderma Lucidum* in Chronic Fatigue Syndrome," *JAASP* 2 (2013): 262–268, https://www.aaspjournal.org/uploads/155/5940_pdf.pdf.

9. Jia Meng and Baoxue Yang, "Protective Effects of Ganoderma (Lingzhi) on Cardiovascular System," *Advances in Experimental Medicine and Biology* 1182 (2019): 181–199, https://pubmed.ncbi.nlm.nih.gov/31777019/.

10. Chiu et al., "Triterpenoids and Polysaccharide Peptides-Enriched *Ganoderma Lucidum*: A Randomized, Double-Blind Placebo-Controlled Crossover Study of Its Antioxidation and Hepatoprotective Efficacy in Healthy Volunteers," *Pharmaceutical Biology* 55, no. 1 (December 2017): 1041–1046, https://pubmed.ncbi.nlm.nih.gov/28183232/.

11. N. Bhardwaj, P. Katyal, A. Sharma, "Suppression of Inflammatory and Allergic Responses by Pharmacologically Potent Fungus *Ganoderma Lucidum*," *Recent Patents on Inflammation & Allergy Drug Discovery* 8, no. 2 (2014): 104–17, https://pubmed.ncbi.nlm.nih.gov/24948193/.

12. Shi et al., "Immunomodulatory Effect of Ganoderma Lucidum Polysaccharides (GLP) on Long-Term Heavy-Load Exercising Mice," *International Journal for Vitamin and Nutrition Research* 82, no. 6 (December 2012): 383–90, https://pubmed.ncbi.nlm.nih.gov/23823923/.

13. Jin et al., "Ganoderma Lucidum (Reishi Mushroom) for Cancer Treatment," *Cochrane Reviews* 13, no 6. (June 2012): CD007731, https://pubmed.ncbi.nlm.nih.gov/22696372/.

14. Martin Powell, "The Use of *Ganoderma Lucidum* (Reishi) in the Management of Histamine-Mediated Allergic Responses," *Townsend Letter: The Examiner of Alternative Medicine* 273 (May 2006) https://www.mycologyresearch.com/articles/view/28.

15. Wu et al., "Evaluation on Quality Consistency of *Ganoderma Lucidum* Dietary Supplements Collected in the United States," *Scientific Reports* 7 (August 2017): 7792, https://www.nature.com/articles/s41598-017-06336-3.

16. Amir A 'lam Kamyab and Ahad Eshraghian, "Anti-Inflammatory, Gastrointestinal and Hepatoprotective Effects of Ocimum Sanctum Linn: An Ancient Remedy with New Application," *Inflammation & Allergy - Drug Targets* 12, no. 6 (December 2013): 378–84, https://pubmed.ncbi.nlm.nih.gov/24266685/.

17. Marc Maurice Cohen, "Tulsi – *Ocimum Sanctum:* A Herb for All Reasons," *Journal of Ayurveda and Integrative Medicine* 5, no. 4 (October–December 2014): 251–259, https://www.ncbi.nlm.nih.gov/pmc/articles/PMC4296439/.

18. Richard et al., "Anti-Stress Activity of Ocimum Sanctum: Possible Effects on Hypothalamic–Pituitary–Adrenal Axis," *Phytotherapy Research* 30, no. 5 (May 2016): 805–14, https://pubmed.ncbi.nlm.nih.gov/26899341/.

19. Bhattacharyya et al., "Controlled Programmed Trial of Ocimum Sanctum Leaf on Generalized Anxiety Disorders," *Nepal Medical College Journal* 10, no. 3 (September 2008): 176–9, https://pubmed.ncbi.nlm.nih.gov/19253862/.

20. P. Prakash and N. Gupta, "Therapeutic Uses of *Ocimum Sanctum* Linn (Tulsi) with a Note of Eugenol and Its Pharmacological Actions: A Short Review,"

Indian Journal of Physiology and Pharmacology 49, no. 2 (April 2005): 125–31, https://pubmed.ncbi.nlm.nih.gov/16170979/.

21. Kamyab et al., "Anti-Inflammatory, Gastrointestinal and Hepaprotective Effects," 378–84.

22. Mondal et al., "Double-Blinded Randomized Controlled Trial for Immunomodulatory Effects on Tulsi (*Ocimum Sanctum* Linn.) Leaf Extract on Healthy Volunteers," *Journal of Ethnopharmacology* 136, no. 3 (July 2011): 452–6, https://pubmed.ncbi.nlm.nih.gov/21619917/.

23. Baliga et al., "Ocimum Sanctum L (Holy Basil or Tulsi) and Its Phytochemicals in the Prevention and Treatment of Cancer," *Nutrition and Cancer* 65, no. Suppl 1 (2013): 26–35, https://pubmed.ncbi.nlm.nih.gov/23682780/.

24. Baliga et al., "Radio Protective Effects of the Ayurvedic Medicinal Plant *Ocium Sanctum* Linn. (Holy Basil): A Memoir," *Journal of Cancer Research and Therapeutics* 12, no. 1 (January–March 2016): 20–7, https://pubmed.ncbi.nlm.nih.gov/27072205/.

25. Moinuddin et al., "Comparative Pharmacological Evaluation of Ocimum Sanctum and Imipramine for Antidepressant Activity," *Latin American Journal of Pharmacy* 30, no. 3 (2011): 435–439, http://sedici.unlp.edu.ar/handle/10915/8159.

26. Chatterjee et al., "Evaluation of Ethanol Leaf Extract of *Ocimum Sanctum* in Experimental Models of Anxiety and Depression," *Pharmaceutical Biology* 49, no. 5 (2011): 477–483, https://www.tandfonline.com/doi/full/10.3109/13880209.2010.523832?journalCode=iphb20.

27. Eleje et al., "Efficacy and Safety of Syferol-IHP for the Treatment of Peptic Ulcer Disease: A Pilot, Double-Blind Randomized Trial," *Clinical and Experimental Gastroenterology* 12 (January 2019): 21–30, https://www.ncbi.nlm.nih.gov/pmc/articles/PMC6338118/.

For Longevity and Well-Being

1. De la Luz Cádiz-Gurrea, "Bioactive Compounds from Theobroma cacao: Effect of Isolation and Safety Evaluation," *Plant Foods for Human Nutrition* 74, no. 1 (March 2019): 40–46, https://pubmed.ncbi.nlm.nih.gov/30324543/.

2. Qais Faryadi, "The Magnificent Effect of Magnesium to Human Health: A Critical Review," *International Journal of Applied Science and Technology* 2, no. 3 (March 2012): 118–126, https://www.dr-qais.com/Qais%20Journal/Magnesium.pdf.

3. Garcia et al., "The Cardiovascular Effects of Chocolate," *Reviews in Cardiovascular Medicine* 19, no. 4 (December 2018): 123–127, https://pubmed.ncbi.nlm.nih.gov/31064163/.

4. D. Katz, K. Doughty, and A. Ali, "Cocoa and Chocolate in Human Health and Disease," *Antioxidants & Redox Signaling* 15, no. 10 (November 2011): 2779–811, https://pubmed.ncbi.nlm.nih.gov/21470061/.

5.   Kamei et al., "Anti-Influenza Virus Effects of Cocoa," *Journal of the Science of Food and Agriculture* 96, no. 4 (March 2016): 1150–8, https://pubmed.ncbi.nlm.nih.gov/25847473/.

6.   Yoneda et al., "Theobromine Up-Regulates Cerebral Brain-Derived Neurotrophic Factor and Facilitates Motor Learning in Mice," *The Journal of Nutritional Biochemistry* 39 (January 2017): 110–116, https://pubmed.ncbi.nlm.nih.gov/27833051/.

7.   Cova et al., "Exploring Cocoa Properties: Is Theobromine a Cognitive Modulator?" *Psychopharmacology* 236, no. 2 (February 2019): 561–572, https://pubmed.ncbi.nlm.nih.gov/30706099/.

8.   Astrid Nehlig, "The Neuroprotective Effects of Cocoa Flavanol and Its Influence on Cognitive Performance," *British Journal of Clinical Pharmacology* 75, no. 3 (March 2013): 716–727, https://www.ncbi.nlm.nih.gov/pmc/articles/PMC3575938/.

9.   Shang et al., "Immunomodulatory and Antioxidant Effects of Polysaccharides from Gynostemma pentaphyllum Makino in Immunosuppressed Mice," *Molecules* 21, no. 8 (August 2016): 1085, https://pubmed.ncbi.nlm.nih.gov/27548135/.

10. Li et al., "Anti-Cancer Effects of *Gynostemma Pentaphyllum* (Thunb.) Makino (*Jiaogulan*)," *Chinese Medicine* 11, no. 43 (September 2016), https://www.ncbi.nlm.nih.gov/pmc/articles/PMC5037898/.

11. Nucific Team, "Gynostemma Pentaphyllum Herb Has Powerful Effects on Health," Nucific, last modified May 31, 2019, https://nucific.com/gynostemma-pentaphyllum/.

12. "Gynostemma," ScienceDirect, last modified 2022, https://www.sciencedirect.com/topics/pharmacology-toxicology-and-pharmaceutical-science/gynostemma.

13. Jia et al., "The Synergistic Effects of Traditional Chinese Herbs and Radiotherapy for Cancer Treatment (Review)," *Oncology Letters* 5, no. 5 (May 2013): 1439–1447, https://www.spandidos-publications.com/10.3892/ol.2013.1245.

14. Huyen et al., "Gynostemma Pentaphyllum Tea Improves Insulin Sensitivity in Type 2 Diabetic Patients," *Journal of Nutrition and Metabolism* 2013 (2013): 765383, https://pubmed.ncbi.nlm.nih.gov/23431428/.

15. Shan Li-Na and Shi Yong-Xi, "Effects of Polysaccharides from Gynostemma Pentaphyllum (Thunb.), Makino on Physical Fatigue," *African Journal of Traditional, Complementary and Alternative Medicine* 11, no. 3 (April 2014): 112–7, https://pubmed.ncbi.nlm.nih.gov/25371572/.

16. Han et al., "The Critical Role of AMPK in Driving Akt Activation Under Stress, Tumorigenesis and Drug Resistance," *Nature Communications* 9, no. 1 (November 2018): 4728, https://pubmed.ncbi.nlm.nih.gov/30413706/.

17. Zhao et al., "ROS Signaling Under Metabolic Stress: Cross-Talk Between AMPK and AKT Pathway," *Molecular Cancer* 16, no. 1 (April 2017): 79, https://pubmed.ncbi.nlm.nih.gov/28407774/.

18. Daniel Garcia and Reuben Shaw, "AMPK: Mechanisms of Cellular Energy Sensing and Restoration of Metabolic Balance," *Molecular Cell* 66, no. 6 (June 2017): 789–800, https://pubmed.ncbi.nlm.nih.gov/28622524/.

19. Townsend et al., "AMPK Mediates Energetic Stress-Induced Liver GDF15," *The FASEB Journal* 35, no. 1 (January 2021): e21218, https://pubmed.ncbi.nlm.nih.gov/33337559/.

20. Choi et al., "Supplementation with Extract of Gynostemma Pentaphyllum Leaves Reduces Anxiety in Healthy Subjects with Chronic Psychological Stress: A Randomized, Double-Blind, Placebo-Controlled Clinical Trial," *Phytomedicine* 52 (January 2019): 198–205, https://pubmed.ncbi.nlm.nih.gov/30599899/.

21. Okoye et al., "18 – Safe African Medicinal Plants for Clinical Studies," *Toxicological Survey of African Medicinal Plants* (2014): 535–555, https://www.sciencedirect.com/science/article/pii/B9780128000182000182.

22. "Moringa's Origins and History," *"Moringa": The Miracle Tree: Food Supplement (Complement Nutritionnel)* (blog). https://superfoodmoringa.blogspot.com/2013/01/moringas-origins-and-history.html.

23. H. Khaliq, Z. Juming, and P. Ke-Mei, "The Physiological Role of Boron on Health," *Biological Trace Element Research* 186, no. 1 (November 2018): 31–51, https://pubmed.ncbi.nlm.nih.gov/29546541/.

24. Vergara-Jimenez, "Bioactive Components in Moringa Oleifera Leaves Protect against Chronic Disease," *Antioxidants* 6, no. 4 (November 2017): 91, https://pubmed.ncbi.nlm.nih.gov/29144438/.

25. Kaur, "Evaluation of the Antidepressant Activity of *Moringa Oleifera* Alone and in Combination with Fluoxetine," *Journal of Ayurveda and Integrative Medicine* 6, no. 4 (October–December 2015): 273–279, https://www.ncbi.nlm.nih.gov/pmc/articles/PMC4719488/.

26. Sun et al., "Effects of Moringa Oleifera Leaves as a Substitute for Alfalfa Meal on Nutrient Digestibility, Growth Performance, Carcass Trait, Meat Quality, Antioxidant Capacity and Biochemical Parameters of Rabbits," *Journal of Animal Physiology and Animal Nutrition* 102, no. 1 (February 2018): 194–203, https://pubmed.ncbi.nlm.nih.gov/28603877/.

27. Minaiyan et al., "Anti-Inflammatory Effect of *Moringa Oleifera* Lam. Seeds on Acetic Acid-Inuced Acute Colitis in Rats," *Avicenna Journal of Phytomedicine* 4, no. 2 (March–April 2014): 127–136, https://www.ncbi.nlm.nih.gov/pmc/articles/PMC4103706/.

28. Rasha Abbas and Fatma Seleman Elsharbasy, "Antibacterial Activity of Moringa Oleifera Against Pathogenic," *International Journal of Current Research* 11, no. 1 (January 2019): 27–30, https://www.researchgate.net/publication/335516212_ANTIBACTERIAL_ACTIVITY_OF_MORINGA_OLEIFERA_AGAINST_PATHOGENIC.

29. Divya et al., "Role of Diet in Dermatological Conditions," *Journal of Nutrition & Food Sciences* 5, no. 5 (2015), https://www.longdom.org/open-access/role-of-diet-in-dermatological-conditions-2155-9600-1000400.pdf.

30. Zawn Villines, "What Are the Benefits of Vitamin E for the Skin?" *MedicalNewsToday*, Healthline Media, last modified April 27, 2021, https://www.medicalnewstoday.com/articles/vitamin-e-for-skin#benefits.

31. De Saint Sauveur and Mélanie Broin, *Growing and Processing Moringa Leaves*, (NA: Moringanews). http://www.moringanews.org/documents/moringawebEN.pdf.

32. Jerry Shay and Woodring Wright, "Role of Telomeres and Telomerase in Cancer," *Seminars in Cancer Biology* 21, no. 6 (June 2012): 349–353, https://www.ncbi.nlm.nih.gov/pmc/articles/PMC3370415/.

33. Tsoukalas et al., "Discovery of Potent Telomerase Activators: Unfolding New Therapeutic and Anti-Aging Perspectives," *Molecular Medicine Reports* 20, no. 4 (October 2019): 3701–3708, https://www.ncbi.nlm.nih.gov/pmc/articles/PMC6755196/.

34. Koehler et al., "The Role of Endophytic/Epiphytic Bacterial Constituents in the Immunostimulatory Activity of the Botanical, *Astragalus Membranaceus*, *Yale Journal of Biology and Medicine* 93, no. 2 (June 2020): 239–250, https://www.ncbi.nlm.nih.gov/pmc/articles/PMC7309664/.

35. Kong et al., "The Current Application and Future Prospects of Astragalus Polysaccharide Combinde with Cancer Immunotherapy: A Review," *Frontiers in Pharmacology* 12 (October 2021): 737674, https://pubmed.ncbi.nlm.nih.gov/34721026/.

36. Meng et al., "Effect of Astragalosides on Intracellular Calcium Overload in Cultured Cardiac Myocytes of Neonatal Rats," *The American Journal of Chinese Medicine* 33, no. 1 (2005): 11–20, https://pubmed.ncbi.nlm.nih.gov/15844829/.

37. Yeh et al., "*Astragalus Membranaceus* Improves Exercise Performance and Ameliorates Exercise-Induced Fatigue in Trained Mice," *Molecules* 19, no. 3 (March 2014): 2793–2807, https://www.ncbi.nlm.nih.gov/pmc/articles/PMC6271379/.

38. Che et al., "Effects of Astragalus Membranaceus Fiber on Growth Performance, Nutrient Digestibility, Microbial Composition, VFA Production, Gut pH, and Immunity of Weaned Pigs," *MicrobiologyOpen* 8, no. 5 (May 2019): e00712, https://www.ncbi.nlm.nih.gov/pmc/articles/PMC6528644/.

PART III

Shopping List

1. Skye Chilton, "74% of Reishi Products Are Not Authentic," RealMushrooms, accessed February 18, 2022, https://www.realmushrooms.com/usp-say-Reishi-products-not-authentic/.

2. https://www.fda.gov/regulatory-information/search-fda-guidance-documents/cpg-sec-585525-mushroom-mycelium-fitness-food-labeling

Creating Your Routine

1. "Corrigent," *The Free Dictionary*, Farlex, accessed February 18, 2022, https://medical-dictionary.thefreedictionary.com/corrigent.

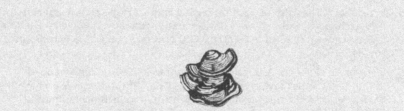

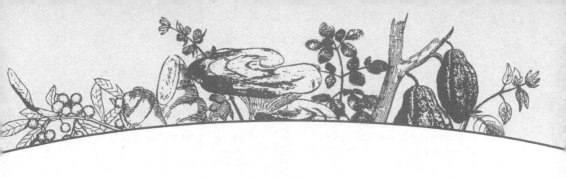

INDEX

Note: Page numbers in **bold** indicate fun fact box overviews of each Adaptogen. Page numbers in *italics* indicate recipes.

Betulinic acid, 41, 42

Bioavailability, ensuring, 179–180

Bodily systems. *See* Systems of your body

Body type
Ayurvedic doshas (vata, pitta, kapha) and, 6, 8–9, 10
energetics and matching medicine to imbalances and, 8–11
TCM constitutions and, 9–11

Brahmi ("creative forces of the earth"). *See* Gotu Kola

Brain and focus
about: case study (Lion's Mane), 105
Ashwagandha helpful for, 129–130, 131
Cacao helpful for, 149–150, 151
Eleuthero helpful for, 49
Ginseng helpful for, 85, 87
Gotu Kola helpful for, 115–116, 118
Lion's Mane helpful for, 101–102, 105
Morning Coffee Recipe for Brain and Performance, *124*
Mucuna helpful for, 108–109, 112
Rhodiola helpful for, 121, 123

Brekhman, Dr. Israel, 12

Broida, Danielle Ryan, about, xv–xvi, 228

Buying Adaptogens. *See* Shopping guide

C

Cacao, **146**–151
about: fun fact summary (full legal name; nicknames; power hub; home; energetics; areas helpful with/common uses; best friends), **146**
brief history of, 147–148
case study, 151
as currency, 147
dosage, 150
Evening Hot Chocolate Recipe for Sleep and Relaxation, *171*
helpful for brain, 149–150, 151
helpful with immunity, 148–149, 151

helpful with longevity, 148, 151
preparation and sourcing, 150
real-life ways to benefit from, 151
for stress, 151

Cancer
about: case study, 45; flavonoids and, 28; phenolic acids and, 28; radioprotector, 154
Acerola and, 76, 77
Astragalus and, 166, 167
Chaga and, 39–40, 41, 45
Ginseng and recovery from, 84
Gotu Kola and, 115
Gynostemma and, 153, 154
Lion's Mane and, 101
Moringa and, 159, 160
Reishi and, 136
Tulsi and, 140, 142, 143
Turkey Tail and, 52–53, 55
Turmeric and, 60

Cancer fungus. *See* Chaga

The Cancer Ward (Solzhenitsyn), 39

Case studies
for brain and focus (Lion's Mane), 105
for energy and performance (Cordyceps), 93
for immunity and protection (Chaga for cancer), 45
for longevity, 151
for stress and mood (Ashwagandha), 131
for stress and mood (Cacao), 151

Caterpillar fungus. *See* Cordyceps

"Ceiling dose," 3

Chaga, **38**–45
about: fun fact summary (full legal name; nicknames; power hub; home; energetics; areas helpful with/common uses; best friends), **38**
brewed as coffee substitute, 39
brief history of, 39
cancer and, 39–40, 41, 45
case study, 45
dosage, 44
extraction process, 43–44
helpful with beauty and skin, 41–42, 45, *79*

H

I

Immune system. *See also* Defend,
    Adaptogens to
Adaptogens supporting, 18
digestive system and, 18–19
immunomodulation (cruise con-
    trol) of, 18
mushrooms as immunomodulators,
    18
as one of 11 body systems, 24
Immunity and protection
    about: activating innate immunity,
        47; case study (Chaga for cancer),
        45; cytokines and, 60, 61, 136,
        141
    Acerola helpful with, 76–77, 79
    Astragalus helpful with, 168–169,
        170
    Cacao helpful with, 148–149, 151
    Chaga helpful with, 39–40, 45
    Eleuthero helpful with, 47–48, 50
    Goji helpful with, 66–67, 68
    Lion's Mane helpful with, 103, 105
    Reishi helpful with, 136–137, 138
    Turkey Tail helpful with, 53, 56
    Turmeric helpful with, 60, 62
Incomparable one. *See* Tulsi
Indian Ginseng. *See* Ashwagandha
Indian saffron. *See* Turmeric
Infertility. *See* Libido
Inflammation
    about: flavonoids for, 28; phenolic
        acids for, 28; polyphenols for,
        28–29; triterpenes for, 27
    Acerola and, 76
    Astragalus and, 168
    Chaga and, 41
    Gynostemma and, 153, 154
    Moringa and, 159, 161, 163
    Reishi and, 136
    Tulsi and, 141, 142, 143
    Turkey Tail and, 54
    Turmeric and, 59, 60, 61, 63
Integumentary system, Adaptogens
    and, 24
Isokauppila, Tero, about, xiv–xv, 227

K

Kakaw. *See* Cacao
Kapha (earth) dosha, 9
Kapikacchu. *See* Mucuna
King of mushrooms. *See* Chaga
Korean Ginseng. *See* Ginseng

L

L-dopa, 108, 109, 110, 111
Lazarev, Dr. Nikolai, 11–12
Li Ching-Yuen, 65
Li Shih-chen, 135
Libido
    about: aphrodisiacs and, 52, 83, 85,
        107, 109–110, 127; blood flow
        and, 19; HGH and, 66, 127–128
    Adaptogens improving, 20, 24
    Ashwagandha and, 128
    Cordyceps helpful with, 89, 91–92,
        93
    Ginseng helpful with, 83, 85, 86, 87
    Goji helpful with, 67, 68
    Maca helpful with, 96–97, 98
    Mucuna helpful with, 109–110, 112
Lingzhi. *See* Reishi
Lion's Mane, **100**–105
    about: fun fact summary (full legal
        name; nicknames; power hub;
        home; energetics; areas helpful
        with/common uses; best friends),
        100
    brief history of, 101
    cancer and, 101
    case study, 105
    dosage, 104
    helpful for brain, 101–102, 105
    helpful with immunity, 103, 105
    helpful with longevity, 102–103,
        105
    Morning Coffee Recipe for Brain
        and Performance, *124*
    nerve growth factors (NGF) and,
        102, 103
    preparation and sourcing, 104
    real-life ways to benefit from, 105
Locoweed. *See* Astragalus
Longevity and well-being

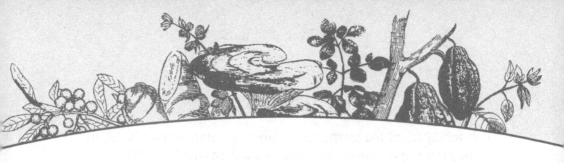

ACKNOWLEDGMENTS

FROM TERO

I would like to acknowledge all my wise ancestors and the preceding 12 generations of the Isokauppila family farm. My mother, Pirkko, my father, Markku, and my brother, Vesa, all have contributed greatly towards who I am today. My loving wife, Cora, and our kids are the greatest thing in my life today! Writing a book while having a young family and fast-growing functional food start-up would not have been possible without my family's support.

I would also like to acknowledge the team that brough this book to life. My book agent, Byrd, and the team at United Talent Agency. All the awesome folks at Hay House—Reid, Allison, Lisa, Tricia and everyone else. Nicola for reading the early version. My business partners, Mikael and Markus. Elizabeth Jarrard for helping out with the book edits. Juho for again making beautiful art for my book. What's the fourth book we will work together on? Most importantly, huge thanks to my awesome co-author, Danielle! This book would not exist without you. Hope you learned a lot and are proud of what we created.

My heart is full of gratitude towards all the other Adaptogen and Mushroom researchers and educators who have come before us. We're standing on your strong shoulders.

Finally, I would like to thank the big electron! Waaaaw!

FROM DANIELLE

I'm deeply humbled by the opportunity to share in words the ancient intent of the plants and mushrooms in this book. There are countless sentient beings that have supported this path in both large and small ways. So first off, thank you to the Adaptogens in this book for their strength, resilience, and willingness to share their magic and medicine with us.

Beyond the species themselves, I must acknowledge the many ancestors, known and unknown, who have used plant and fungi medicine, paving the way for us to know and use these species today. To all the medicine people who foraged, processed, experimented, and documented their use with these plants and fungi so we could learn and grow from the foundation you laid. My gratitude goes out to the many herbal mentors, instructors, wise-women, and teachers I have had along the way. A special shoutout to my herbal family at the Colorado School of Clinical Herbalism, Lisa, Paul, Kat, Josh, and Lyn. Thank you to my first mushroom teacher, Peter McCoy, for opening my eyes to the fascinating world of fungi. Thanks to our wonderful team at Hay House who has worked behind the scenes to make this book possible.

I would like to acknowledge my partner, Gavin, for the unconditional support and motivation throughout this process. My mother, Julie, and sister, Nicole, for always reminding me of my worth. To Elizabeth, my coworker and partner in crime, who was there along this whole process helping with every logistical detail along the way. Thank you to our brilliant illustrator, Juho, for bringing this book to life through images. And a huge thank you to my co-author, Tero, for proposing we write this book years ago and for making it come to life!

Lastly, my deepest acknowledgment is to this Earth, the place I feel so blessed to call home. The place that provides us with all of the nourishment and medicine we could ever need. I am eternally grateful to each and every life form involved in allowing us to access these healing Adaptogens.

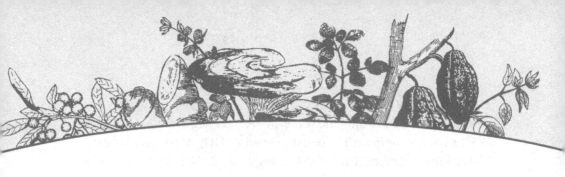

ABOUT THE AUTHORS

TERO ISOKAUPPILA is the founder and CEO of Four Sigmatic, a functional foods company that wants to make the world's most studied and nutrient-dense foods more delicious and easier to consume to bring healthy upgrades into America's daily routine.

Tero's roots (or mycelium, if you will) are in Finland, where he grew up growing and foraging natural foods on his 13th generation family's farm. He later earned a degree in Chemistry, Business, and a Certificate in Plant-Based Nutrition at Cornell University. In 2012, Tero founded Four Sigmatic with the dream of bringing a little Everyday Magic to the lives of all.

An expert in all things related to nutrition, health, and wellness. Tero is the author of two previous best-selling books: *Healing Mushrooms*, an educational cookbook from Avery Publishing, and *Santa Sold Shrooms*, a children's book for adults about the magical origins of Santa Claus.

Tero was chosen twice as one of the world's Top 50 Food Activists by the Academy of Culinary Nutrition and has appeared in *Time*, *Forbes*, BuzzFeed, *Vogue*, *Playboy*, *GQ*, *Harper's Bazaar*, and *Bon Appétit*. He is also a sought-after speaker, featured at Summit Series, Wanderlust, WME-IMG, Google, and the Fast Company Innovation Festival.

Tero splits his time between Austin, Texas and their family farm in Finland.

DANIELLE RYAN BROIDA, RH (AHG), is a key player in the worldwide mushroom movement. As a Registered Herbalist (RH) of the American Herbalists Guild (AHG), Certified Holistic Nutritionist, Instructor of Mycology, and National Educator of Four Sigmatic, Danielle is teaching the world about the importance of life on functional mushrooms.

Prior to joining forces with Four Sigmatic, she received her BA in Environmental Studies and Philosophy from Whitman College. She went on to study Ayurveda in India and became a Certified Yoga Instructor on the banks of the Ganges River. She then worked with a naturopathic doctor in Indonesia, where she became a Certified Raw Chef and Detox Coach. But it was leading trekking adventures into the backcountry of Thailand where she became particularly fascinated by herbal medicine (while also becoming fluent in Thai).

After several years in Asia, she landed in Boulder, Colorado, to formalize her education in holistic medicine. Upon completing her graduate studies at the Colorado School of Clinical Herbalism (CSCH), she opened her private practice, where she worked with hundreds of clients specializing in a functional mushroom-based treatment for individuals with autoimmune conditions and chronic illness. She was invited to become the Instructor of Mycology at CSCH, where she still teaches.

Hay House Titles of Related Interest

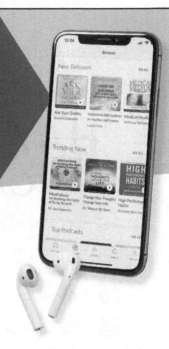

CONNECT WITH
HAY HOUSE
ONLINE

🌐 hayhouse.co.uk   **f** @hayhouse

📷 @hayhouseuk   𝕏 @hayhouseuk

▶ @hayhouseuk   ♪ @hayhouseuk

*Find out all about our latest books & card decks • Be the first
to know about exclusive discounts • Interact with our authors
in live broadcasts • Celebrate the cycle of the seasons with us
• Watch free videos from your favourite authors •
Connect with like-minded souls*

*'The gateways to wisdom and knowledge
are always open.'*

Louise Hay